CASES in
HEALTHCARE
FINANCE

CASES in HEALTHCARE FINANCE

FIFTH EDITION

LOUIS C. GAPENSKI | GEORGE H. PINK

Health Administration Press, Chicago
Association of University Programs in Health Administration, Arlington, Virginia

Your board, staff, or clients may also benefit from this book's insight. For more information on quantity discounts, contact the Health Administration Press Marketing Manager at (312) 424-9470.

18   17   16   15   14   5   4   3   2   1

Gapenski, Louis C.
  Cases in healthcare finance / Louis C. Gapenski, George H. Pink. – Fifth edition.
    pages cm
  ISBN 978-1-56793-611-7 (alk. paper)
  1. Health facilities–Finance–Case studies. 2.   Medical care–Finance–Case studies.   I. Pink, George H. II. Title.
  RA971.3.G367 2013
  362.1068'1–dc23
                        2013026943

The paper used in this publication meets the minimum requirements of American National Standard for Information Sciences—Permanence of Paper for Printed Library Materials, ANSI Z39.48-1984. ∞ ™

Acquisitions editor: Janet Davis; Project manager: Joyce Dunne; Layout: Fine Print, Ltd.; Cover design: Marisa Jackson

Found an error or a typo? We want to know! Please e-mail it to hap1@ache.org, and put "Book Error" in the subject line.

For photocopying and copyright information, please contact Copyright Clearance Center at www.copyright.com or at (978) 750-8400.

Health Administration Press
A division of the Foundation of the American
    College of Healthcare Executives
One North Franklin Street, Suite 1700
Chicago, IL 60606
(312) 424-2800

Association of University Programs
    in Health Administration
2000 North 14th Street,
    Suite 780
Arlington, VA 22201
(703) 894-0940

Contents

Preface for Instructors

HEALTHCARE FINANCE CAN be a fascinating, exciting subject, yet students often regard it as being either too theoretical or too mechanical. The fact is, sound financial decision making requires good theory and analysis plus a great deal of insight and judgment. The best way to get this point across to students, and to demonstrate the inherent richness of the subject, is to relate classroom work to real-world decision making. When this is done, students must grapple not only with the concepts but also, and more important, with how the concepts are applied in practice.

Of course, the most realistic application of healthcare finance occurs within healthcare organizations, and there is no substitute for on-the-job experience. The next best thing, and the only real option for the classroom, is to use cases to simulate the environment in which financial decisions are made.

Purpose

The purpose of this casebook is to provide students with an opportunity to bridge the gap between learning concepts in a classroom setting and actually applying them in the real world. By using these cases, instructors can help students who have a basic understanding of healthcare finance better prepare for the multitude of problems that arise in practice.

Content

This casebook consists of 32 cases, which focus on healthcare finance issues, and seven mini-cases, which focus on ethical issues related to healthcare finance. In general, each finance case addresses a single issue, such as capital budgeting analysis or revenue cycle management, but the uncertainty of the input data, along with the presence of relevant nonfinancial factors, makes each case interesting and challenging. Because the finance cases focus on both accounting and financial management decisions, they cover the full range of health-care finance. Furthermore, the case settings include a wide variety of organizational settings, including hospitals, clinics, medical practices, home health care organizations, integrated delivery systems, and managed care organizations.

Each ethics mini-case contains a very short description of a finance situation that has potential ethical implications. These cases require no numerical analysis; rather, they are intended to be used as discussion vehicles for healthcare finance instructors who want to include finance-related ethics content in their courses.

Directed Versus Nondirected Cases

In general, cases may be classified as directed or nondirected. Directed cases include a specific set of questions that students must answer to complete the case, while nondirected cases (as we use the term) contain only general guidance to point students in the right direction. The cases in this book are nondirected. The primary advantage of nondirected cases is that they closely resemble how real-world managers confront financial decision making because the cases require students to develop their own solution approach. The disadvantage is that students who stray from the key issues of the cases often do not obtain full value from their effort.

In general, students with more advanced analytical and logic skills and relevant work experience gain the most from nondirected cases, while students who have had less exposure to casework and little or no work experience gain the most from directed cases. The online Instructor's Resources for this casebook contain a set of case questions for each case that can be given to students to convert these cases into directed cases. Thus, instructors have the option of using the cases in either way, depending on the experience of the students, the objectives of the course, and the extent to which cases will be used.

Using This Casebook

The cases can be used in several different ways. For example, the case-book is the foundation for the second healthcare finance course in the University of Florida's MHA program. Students in this program take an introductory healthcare finance course that includes both accounting and financial management basics; the second course focuses on the application of finance concepts within health services organizations.

The course is essentially a pure case course, and about 15 cases (one per week) are assigned. The students have had sufficient lecture work in healthcare finance, so at this stage learning by doing is the best way to prepare them for success in their chosen field. The students are not provided with the accompanying case questions, so they must develop their own approaches to completing each case.

A team of four or five students is assigned to present each case in class. Teams that are not presenting must turn in written reports and act as members of the board of directors during the presentation. They are responsible for asking relevant questions of the presenting team and pointing out any deficiencies in the analysis. Group work provides excellent experience for students because almost all decision making in business is done in a group environment, and individuals who cannot work in groups are doomed to failure. Students will need to know how to motivate the people who work for them and be able to work with others in a cooperative manner. An in-class presentation also provides students the opportunity to hone their presentation skills. Healthcare executives constantly state that the ability to communicate is absolutely critical to success in business. We agree. Knowledge of healthcare finance (or any other managerial discipline) is useless unless the individual can communicate his or her ideas to others.

In addition to their use in a pure case course, the cases can be used in other ways. For example, the MHA program at the University of North Carolina at Chapel Hill offers two second-year healthcare finance courses. The first course covers basic financial management concepts, capital acquisition, cost of capital, and capital structure. The second course covers capital allocation, financial condition analysis and forecasting, and other topics. Each course includes six to seven cases, which the students either present or discuss in class as guided by the instructor.

Finally, we find that the cases work particularly well in executive MHA programs. Executive students generally bring a great deal of real-world insights into their case analyses, which often makes the discussions livelier than those in traditional programs. In addition, the cases can be worked during the intervals between on-campus sessions, which allows plenty of time for group discussion and analysis.

Spreadsheet Models

Spreadsheet analysis has become extremely important in all aspects of healthcare finance, so the cases have accompanying models that allow students to hone and improve their spreadsheet skills. Furthermore, spreadsheet models can reduce the amount of busywork required to perform analyses and hence leave students with more time to focus on finance issues as well as qualitative factors that are relevant to the decision at hand.

To facilitate spreadsheet use, we developed well-structured, user-friendly models for each case. The spreadsheet models are efficient and hence big time savers, especially when conducting risk assessment using techniques such as sensitivity and scenario analyses. In addition, spreadsheet models allow students to easily create graphics and other spreadsheet output that enhance the quality of both the analyses and the presentations.

As we considered students' use of these models, an important question arose: Should we provide complete models to students, or should students be required to do some (or all) of the modeling themselves? After testing several different approaches, we concluded that the best solution for most cases is to provide students with complete versions of the case models such that no modeling is required to obtain a base case solution. However, zeros have been entered for all input data in the student versions, and hence students must identify and then enter the appropriate input data. When this is done, the model automatically calculates the base case solution. However, the models do not contain risk analyses or other extensions such as graphics, so students must modify the models as necessary to make them most useful in completing the cases. The student versions of the case models can be accessed through the Health Administration Press website at ache.org/books/FinanceCases5. Students should visit the site to download the student version models. (Note that there are no student models for the cases under Financial Management Basics [Cases 12–15] because these concepts are best learned when students must do their own calculations.)

In addition to the student versions of the spreadsheet models for 28 cases, there are instructor versions for all 32 finance cases. These differ from the student models primarily because the input data are intact in the instructor versions.

Changes in the Fifth Edition

We have used the fourth edition in numerous courses since its publication and have benefited from many student comments and suggestions. Moreover, we have received suggestions from other instructors in different settings. This feedback has resulted in many changes, both substantial and minor.

The most substantial change to the casebook involves authorship. While the fourth edition was written in collaboration with George H. Pink, a professor of health policy and management at the University of North Carolina at Chapel Hill, in this edition George participates as a coauthor. As many of you know, George also is the coauthor of the sixth edition of *Understanding Healthcare Financial Management*, the book that often is used as an accompanying textbook to this casebook. George brings many new insights to the cases, which continue to have a profound and positive impact on the book.

Many minor changes have been made to improve the cases and accompanying material. For example, the names were changed on all cases, and recent changes in the health services environment have been incorporated to ensure the cases remain contemporary. In addition, specific questions that were embedded in the case prose have been removed to allow instructors to have more influence over the amount of direction given to students. The case questions (available to instructors for distribution to students if desired) have been revised to focus on more complex calculation and interpretation issues rather than on definitional and background issues. In addition, the last question in each case now asks students to identify three key learning points. Our primary goal in making these changes was to improve the pedagogic value of the cases. In addition, in most cases without major changes, we altered a number or two so that the solutions changed slightly. This was done to invalidate the old "fraternity files" that might be passed from one cohort to the next. Still, we did not want to change the underlying character of the cases because (1) they work well now, and (2) we do not want instructors to have to relearn the cases each time a new edition is published.

Regarding ancillary materials, the case slideshows have been substantially changed. Instead of a review of the accounting or financial management concepts relevant to the case, the slideshows now are intended to be used solely as a case introduction (for presentation before student analysis) and a case conclusion (for presentation after student analysis) that focuses on three key learning points.

The spreadsheet models have been reviewed for computational accuracy and ease of use with changes made as needed. Additionally, four new models were created so every case now has an instructor's spreadsheet model. These new instructor's models (for the Financial Management Basics cases [12–15]) make the calculations fully transparent to the instructor and aid in answering student questions. However, there are no student models for these cases, so students still must perform the required calculations using either a financial calculator or a spreadsheet model that they create.

In addition to these relatively minor changes, some of the cases have been changed more substantially. Here is a listing of those cases with a brief summary of the changes, which have been classified as either extensive or moderate.

Case 1: River Community Hospital (A). This hospital financial performance assessment case has been revised extensively. There are three years of data, instead of five; an exhibit has been added; the instructor's spreadsheet has new summary tables that show where the hospital is better or worse than industry benchmarks and where this year's performance is better or worse than last year's performance; and there are new calculation and interpretation questions.

Case 8: Mountain Village Clinic. This cash budgeting case has been revised moderately. Students are asked to create a cash budget for a "worst case scenario," and there are new calculation and interpretation questions.

Case 12: Gulf Shores Surgery Centers. This time value analysis case has been revised extensively. The case prose has been rewritten to focus on four practical time value problems, an exhibit has been added, and all of the calculation questions have been rewritten.

Case 13: Mid-Atlantic Specialty, Inc. This financial risk case has been revised extensively. The case prose has been rewritten to focus on calculation and application of stand-alone, corporate, and market risk measures; an exhibit has been added; and there are new calculation and interpretation questions.

Case 14: Pacific Healthcare (A). This bond valuation case has been revised extensively. The case prose has been rewritten to focus on valuation, yields, and risk; an exhibit has been added; and there are new calculation and interpretation questions.

Case 15: Pacific Healthcare (B). This stock valuation case has been revised extensively. The case prose has been rewritten to focus on current and future stock valuation and yields, an exhibit has been added, and there are new calculation and interpretation questions.

Case 16: Senior Care Enterprises. This bond refunding case has been revised extensively. The case prose has been rewritten to focus on three bond-refunding options, the effects of interest rates and tax rates on the refunding decision are emphasized, the replacement chain analysis has been deleted, and there are new calculation and interpretation questions.

Case 17: Seattle Cancer Center. This leasing decisions case has been revised moderately. A volume/profit graphic has been added to the instructor spreadsheet, and there are new calculation and interpretation questions.

Case 18: Southeastern Homecare. This corporate cost of capital case has been revised extensively. The case prose has been rewritten to focus on factors that affect the corporate cost of capital, application of divisional costs of capital, not-for-profit cost of capital, and use of weights; an exhibit has been added; and there are new calculation and interpretation questions.

Case 19: RN Temps, Inc. This capital structure analysis case has been revised extensively. The case prose has been rewritten to focus on the effects of financial leverage on return on equity, stock price, corporate cost of capital, and business risk, and there are new calculation and interpretation questions.

Case 20: Coral Bay Hospital. This traditional project analysis case has been revised moderately. There are new calculation and interpretation questions.

Case 25: Bedford Clinics. This practice valuation case has been revised extensively. The case prose has been rewritten to focus on acquisition of a practice by a large system; another market multiple (EBITDA, or earnings before interest, taxes, depreciation, and amortization) has been added; analysis is now required to select values for market multiples; an exhibit has been added; and there are new calculation and interpretation questions.

Finally, two new finance cases and one ethics mini-case have been added to the book.

Case 16: Senior Care Enterprises. This bond refunding case (see description above) was previously available online. It is now included in the casebook.

Case 30: Milwaukee Regional Health System. This revenue cycle management case, coauthored with Scott Hawig, focuses on the very important topics of revenue cycle management and chargemaster pricing.

Ethics Mini-Case 7: Spotlight on PODs. This physician-owned distributorships mini-case focuses on the potential ethical conflicts involved in PODs.

We are convinced that these changes will make the casebook even more useful for instructors and more beneficial for students in their quest for competency in healthcare finance.

Instructor's Resources

The following teaching aids are available for instructors who adopt this casebook:

- *PowerPoint slides.* Each case is accompanied by a short slideshow that first introduces the main features of the case and model and then wraps up the case with three key learning points. Instructors may either use these slides as is or customize them to meet unique class needs.
- *Case questions.* A set of questions for each case is available for those instructors who want to convert the cases from nondirected to directed format.
- *Case solutions.* Each case has a comprehensive solution that is based on the case questions.
- *Instructor models.* The instructor's version of each case spreadsheet model can be downloaded from the Instructor Resources web page through the "In the Classroom" link. (Note that a password is required to access the Instructor Resources.) This model is similar to the student model except that the input values are intact. Thus, instructors can view the base case solution without entering any data. In addition, some instructor versions include additional modeling, such as risk analyses.

Acknowledgments

This casebook reflects the efforts of many people besides the primary authors. First, several of the cases that appear in this and previous editions were coauthored by the following individuals:

- Murray Côté
- Robert Harmon
- Ian Jamieson
- Brett Justice
- Paul Phillips

In addition, Case 30 (Milwaukee Regional Health System) is coauthored by Scott Hawig, senior vice president of finance at Froedtert Health in Milwaukee, Wisconsin.

Finally, colleagues, students, and staff provided inspirational support, as well as more tangible support, during the development and class testing of the revised cases. In addition, the Health Administration Press staff was instrumental in ensuring the quality and usefulness of this casebook.

Conclusion

The field of healthcare finance continues to undergo significant changes and advances. Participating in these developments is stimulating, and we sincerely hope that the fifth edition of *Cases in Healthcare Finance* helps students gain a better appreciation for the application of finance principles to healthcare organizations.

A book that raises so many issues will also inevitably generate a variety of opinions regarding both financial theory and practice. Furthermore, although both the publisher and the authors have placed great emphasis on the accuracy of the cases and accompanying materials, some discrepancies or inconsistencies may exist. We appreciate any comments, corrections, criticisms, and ideas for improving all aspects of the cases and related materials.

Professor Louis C. Gapenski, PhD
Department of Health Services Research, Management and Policy
Box 100195, Health Science Center
University of Florida
Gainesville, FL 32610-0195
E-mail: gapenski@ufl.edu

George H. Pink, PhD
Humana Distinguished Professor
Department of Health Policy and Management
University of North Carolina at Chapel Hill
1105D McGavran-Greenberg Hall CB 7411
Chapel Hill, NC 27599
E-mail: gpink@email.unc.edu

Preface for Students

THERE IS NO better way to learn healthcare finance than by working cases. Of course, it is necessary first to have a basic understanding of the principles and concepts that will be applied in the cases, and this knowledge generally is obtained from previous classroom work.

The finance cases in this book present situations that require analysis and judgment regarding financial decision making. Although the emphasis here is on financial analysis, real-world decisions are based as much (perhaps more) on qualitative factors as on the numbers. This means that you must consider not only the financial implications of the cases but also the relevant nonfinancial considerations before reaching final conclusions and making recommendations.

Working the Cases

All finance cases, except the Financial Management Basics cases (12–15), have accompanying spreadsheet models. These models can be downloaded from the Health Administration Press website at ache.org/books/FinanceCases5. Note that the input data in these models have been zeroed out. Thus, you will have to enter the appropriate values for these data to get the models to "work." Also, note that the models contain only base case analyses. You must add to the models any extensions required by the case, such as risk analyses and graphics (charts).

Note that for most cases there is more than one right answer. Indeed, in some cases, multiple approaches to the solution may be appropriate. The critical issue in presenting your findings is your ability to support your conclusions and recommendations.

An unlimited number of approaches to working cases exist, and the approach that is optimal for one individual (or group) is not necessarily the best for another individual (or group). That said, here are some suggested steps to help in your casework. (Note that the cases differ in content, and hence one size [the steps below] does not fit all. Also, note that the guidance given here is generic in nature and does not take precedence over the guidance provided by your instructor.)

1. Scan the case to get an overall idea of the setting, topic, and decision at hand.
2. Look at the accompanying spreadsheet model to get a feel for its structure and the nature of the input data needed.
3. Read the case to identify alternative courses of action and to extract the data needed (typically model inputs) for the numerical analysis.
4. Enter the base case data into the spreadsheet model, and check for any problems that might arise, including illogical results.
5. Conduct scenario, sensitivity, and other analyses as needed to either assess risk or make judgments about how uncertainty affects alternative courses of action.
6. Identify the qualitative factors that bear on the decision at hand. Don't forget this step!
7. Reach your final conclusions, which should logically lead to your recommendations.

Most of the information required to successfully work a case is contained in the case itself. However, you may encounter situations in which additional information would allow you either to feel more comfortable in your recommendations or to examine out-of-the-box solutions. By all means, feel free to pull data from other sources as needed to create a more complete case solution. In fact, if the data needed are not easily available from other sources, there is nothing wrong with making your own assumptions—as long as they pass the "reasonableness" test.

Making a Presentation

Many of you, either as individuals or as a group, will be required to present your case analysis in class. Generally, your audience will not have written material to refer to (except perhaps for supporting financial statements, numerical tables, and so on). Thus, you must structure your presentation so that it can be easily followed and understood the first time around. Although most cases involve a great deal of detailed information, your presentation will be easy to follow if it is simply and clearly organized.

All effective presentations consist of four parts: (1) introduction, (2) body (analysis), (3) conclusions, and (4) recommendations. The first step in preparing a presentation is to construct the body. This is the analysis that must convince the audience that your conclusions and recommendations have merit. If the body is too long and complex, the audience will not be able to grasp its implications and hence will not understand the rationale behind your conclusions and recommendations. Conversely, an analysis that is too short will appear to be lacking in thought and substance and will raise more questions than it will provide answers. Similarly, a body that is not presented in a step-wise, logical sequence may contain the right information but still not get the job done because the audience just can't follow its logic.

Once the body of the presentation has been prepared, the introduction, conclusions, and recommendations should be added. The introduction serves three purposes: (1) gain the audience's attention, (2) describe the decision at hand, and (3) preview the main ideas that will be covered in the remainder of the presentation.

A presentation can have an excellent introduction and body, but it may still be totally ineffective. There is nothing worse than a presentation that trails off "into the sunset," leaving the audience in the dark as to why they just spent 30 minutes listening. The conclusions must be strong and convincing such that the audience recognizes that a sound and thorough analysis has been achieved. Finally, the recommendations must provide concrete suggestions for action. In essence, the conclusions and recommendations should provide closure for the audience. Any questions remaining at this point should involve technical details as opposed to "What did you say we should do?"

Preparing the Slides

In most cases, you will be using PowerPoint slides as the basis for the presentations. Don't forget that the primary function of slides is to support your message. Thus, the slides must contain the key elements of the introduction, body (analysis), conclusions, and recommendations. Slides that are irrelevant or confusing detract from the presentation. Also, too many slides is just as confusing to the audience as too few slides.

Don't try to put a great deal of numerical detail on slides. For example, several years of financial statements on a single slide will not be readable to the audience. Similarly, breaking the statements into sections so that they are on multiple slides is a poor idea, because the audience will not be able to see all the data at one time. For large amounts of data, handouts are preferable to slides. The key points should be on slides, but use handouts to provide the audience with numerical details.

Working in Groups

Many of you will be working in groups. For some students, this is a blessing; for others, group work is a curse. The advantage of working in groups is that more talent typically is brought to the table. The disadvantage is that group work can create logistics problems: when the group can meet, what each group member's role is, and so on.

Good groups recognize comparative advantage and capitalize on it. Students who are good at spreadsheets can be the "geek," students who are good at problem solving can be the "brain," students who are good slide makers can be the "artist," and students who are good at verbal communications can be the "face." There is nothing wrong with focusing on individuals' strengths. However, each member of the group is still accountable for all phases of the work. All group members must actively review and approve the work done by other team members. If one member of the group makes a major error, this fact must be noted and corrected by the other members of the group. If a group allows one member to sink the ship, then the entire group is going to drown. Groups in which individuals play different roles do the best casework, but all members ultimately must review and approve the final product.

Some Final Words

When all is said and done, the key to a good case analysis and presentation is preparedness: "Proper prior planning prevents poor performance." This philosophy applies to all phases of casework, including the presentation itself. How many times have you witnessed a presentation that starts 15 minutes late because the laptop or projector doesn't work or one of the presenters is late? Or, midway through the presentation, a slide either is missing or contains typographical errors? Such "small things" cast a shadow of doubt over the analysis and presentation and hence reflect poorly on the entire effort, but they can easily be, and should be, avoided by proper planning.

Case Descriptions

Case 1: This case requires the financial statement analysis of a 210-bed hospital, including financial and operating ratio analysis. The accompanying spreadsheet model does most of the calculations, so students can focus on analysis, interpretation, and recommendations for managerial actions.

Case 2: This is similar to Case 1 in many ways, but it focuses on the managed care industry. It presents two years of data and discusses benchmarking against primary competitors as well as the industry. In spite of structural similarities, the metrics used and the analysis and interpretation are significantly different from Case 1.

Case 3: This case focuses on the question of what constitutes a good cost driver. Students must ponder the "fairness" of allocating a higher amount of facilities overhead to a department that is being forced to move to a new facility. The case raises many issues regarding cost drivers, fairness, and cost-reduction effectiveness.

Case 4: This case focuses on the mathematics of cost allocation. Students must use four allocation methods (direct, step down, double apportionment, and reciprocal) to allocate costs from three support departments to three patient service departments. It is very mechanical in nature and does not require significant consideration of qualitative issues.

Case 5: This case focuses on the development of a premium rate to be offered to a buyer consortium. Students must deal with coverage limitations and copays, as well as the basic costs of providing services. In addition, the case requires the conversion of an aggregate per-member per-month cost into subscriber (single and family) premium rates.

Case 6: This case involves the volume break-even analysis of an unprofitable hospital-owned walk-in clinic. Because the spreadsheet model for this case does the busywork, students can concentrate on the problems inherent in volume break-even analysis and its value to managers in making service decisions. In addition, many qualitative factors play a role in this case.

Case 7: This case focuses on a budgeting variance analysis of four managed care product lines. Because of the large number of required calculations, the accompanying spreadsheet model does the mathematical busywork. To add to the mathematical complexity, the case involves both utilization and enrollment differences. Although the calculations are somewhat mechanical, there is ample room for student interpretation and recommendations.

Case 8: This case is a traditional cash budgeting exercise. It calls for students to develop six monthly budgets, a daily budget for a single month, and a worst case budget. The spreadsheet model, which reduces the amount of busywork required, facilitates sensitivity analyses regarding both patient volume and collection experience. The case presents students with the opportunity to discuss many facets of cash management.

Case 9: This case focuses on the pricing of transplant services. It requires students to do some calculations, but not a large-scale quantitative effort. The primary purpose of the case is to allow students to consider alternative (full versus marginal) pricing approaches when negotiating with third-party payers. It also emphasizes that, in some situations, marginal costs include marginal fixed costs as well as variable costs.

Case 10: This case focuses on using activity based costing (ABC) techniques to estimate the costs associated with two alternative approaches to providing ultrasound services. Although this case is not complex, it allows students to experience the complexities associated with ABC analysis. The case includes sensitivity analyses on many input variables and considers various qualitative factors that affect the selection decision.

Case 11: This case involves the measurement of physician productivity, financial performance, and quality of care and the use of those measures in determining pay for performance. Alternative methodologies are proposed in the case, and students must choose among those given. The case also raises issues about how to ensure that compensation systems can be trusted, understood, equitable, and affordable in addition to providing proper incentives.

Case 12: This case focuses on the mechanics of time value analysis. Because the case is meant to make students think about the time value process and understand the underlying calculations, it does not have an accompanying student spreadsheet model.

Case 13: This case focuses on basic financial risk concepts. Its goal is to give students a sound understanding of the three types of financial risk (stand-alone, corporate, and market) and their implications for decision making within healthcare organizations. Like Case 12, this case has no accompanying student spreadsheet model.

Case 14: This case focuses on the mechanics of bond valuation, as opposed to the managerial decisions inherent in floating a bond issue. This case has no accompanying student spreadsheet model. Here, much of the bond valuation work is at the basic level, but the case includes issues pertaining to yield to call and expected rate of return when an issue has a sinking fund.

Case 15: This case takes students through the mechanics of stock valuation (not the managerial decision process that surrounds a new stock issue), including both the constant and nonconstant growth dividend models. No student spreadsheet model is included.

Case 16: This case focuses on the mechanics of the bond refunding decision. The accompanying spreadsheet model does the mathematical busywork. The case presents three refunding options and asks students to make a specific choice. In addition, several qualitative issues are presented.

Case 17: This case looks at the equipment leasing decisions facing a hospital. The case requires students to perform both lessee's and lessor's analyses. It brings out many side issues, including the correct discount rate, how to deal with residual value uncertainty, the impact of cancelation and per procedure clauses, and the effects on both parties of leveraging the lease.

Case 18: This case focuses on the estimation of a business's cost of capital, including both corporate and divisional costs. Because the required calculations are relatively simple, the accompanying spreadsheet model is very basic. However, students have to grapple with numerous conceptual issues regarding both estimation methodologies and the interpretation and use of the cost of capital once it is estimated.

Case 19: This case examines the capital structure decision for an investor-owned company that franchises "rent-a-nurse" businesses. Here, the primary analytical tool is a zero-growth model that calculates stock price under alternative capital structures. However, the case also examines the impact of financial leverage on accounting profits and asks students to consider the business's value under two theoretical models (Modigliani-Miller and Miller). Also, the case requires students to consider qualitative factors in making the final decision.

Case 20: This case contains a traditional (no nuances) capital budgeting analysis, including cash flow estimation, decision measures, risk assessment, and risk incorporation. In evaluating the financial attractiveness of a proposed outpatient surgery center, students are confronted with many of the problems that occur in such analyses. An accompanying spreadsheet model helps with the calculations. This is a good case for illustrating Monte Carlo simulation.

Case 21: This case focuses on the advantages of making significant capital investments in stages rather than as a large single investment. It uses decision tree methodology to determine project risk and to illustrate the benefits of abandonment. The accompanying spreadsheet model permits students to spend more time on conceptual matters and takes the tedium out of the calculations.

Case 22: This case investigates three alternative proposals for a hospital system's printshop, including closure and outsourcing all work. It also requires students to grapple with several technical issues related to discounted cash flow analysis, such as the handling of non-normal cash flows. Finally, the case examines the strategic issue of entering the commercial (for-profit) printing market.

Case 23: This case explores the valuation of a not-for-profit hospital for possible acquisition by another not-for-profit hospital. In addition to the numerical analysis, the case raises several issues related to control after the merger. Although the accompanying spreadsheet model does the busywork, students must think a great deal about the impact of the merger on both entities and how future cash flows are affected.

Case 24: This case focuses on the analysis of a proposed joint venture involving three equity partners: a hospital and group practice as general partners and individual physicians as limited partners. Students must consider both the costs of capital for the partners and how the partnership cash flows should be allocated across the equity participants. Additionally, the case addresses several qualitative issues, including the risks associated with new, unproven technology and the ethical (and legal) issues involved in income-generating referrals.

Case 25: This case requires students to value a family physician group practice. The case provides data to allow students to use both discounted cash flow and market multiple methodologies. Because of a host of qualitative and quantitative issues, the ultimate "answer" here is filled with uncertainties. More data are given in this case than in Case 22, so fewer assumptions are required. The spreadsheet model helps with the calculations.

Case 26: This case focuses on the use of physician extenders in three clinical settings. Students must make judgments about which type of extender (physician assistant or nurse practitioner) is most appropriate for each clinic. Additionally, students must perform a cost–benefit analysis to assess the financial impact. The spreadsheet model eases the quantitative burden, but students must make the hard assumptions needed regarding extender impact on volumes, reimbursements, and costs.

Case 27: This case focuses on a capital investment decision that involves the use of alternative technologies. To complicate the analysis, one technology frees up inpatient beds for alternative purposes (backfill). The case examines a simplistic replacement analysis, which also makes students consider the differences in replacement versus new project analyses.

Case 28: This case focuses on the basics of receivables management. A start-up drug company is used to illustrate such concepts as average collection period (days sales outstanding), aging schedules, uncollected balances schedules, and the cost of carrying receivables. To complicate matters, these concepts must be applied to multiple customers.

Case 29: This case leads students through an inventory decision process involving supplier selection and optimal ordering quantity (and hence inventory level). The case focuses primarily on the economic ordering quantity model, although students must also categorize inventory items according to the activity based costing model.

Case 30: This case focuses on the revenue cycle management process. Students are required to choose appropriate metrics to measure both overall performance and performance within each revenue cycle function. In addition, students must compare both hospital and clinic metric values against national benchmarks and suggest improvement actions where needed. The case also requires students to calculate and compare chargemaster prices to actual reimbursement amounts for several different payers.

Case 31: This case, which builds on the information given in Case 1, focuses on the development of a hospital's forecasted financial statements. It encompasses both forecasting and financial accounting considerations. Although the accompanying spreadsheet model provides a framework for the forecasting process, students must modify the model to incorporate appropriate forecasting techniques. In addition, students must make an extensive set of assumptions about both the future of the hospital industry and the operations of one particular hospital.

Case 32: This case focuses on the problems faced by a physician–hospital organization (PHO) when one of its most important payers proposes that its fee-for-service payment methodology change to a fixed per-member per-month payment. This situation forces the PHO to consider how to handle a full-risk contract in regard to both utilization risk and how the fixed payment and the associated risk should be shared among the hospital, specialist physicians, and primary care physicians.

Ethics Mini-Cases

Mini-Case 1: This case discusses a situation in which a patient pays a copayment based on full charges (chargemaster prices) while the insurer pays much less than full charges because of contractual discounts.

Mini-Case 2: This case explores the issues associated with corporate ownership (in which the corporation is the beneficiary) of individual life insurance policies.

Mini-Case 3: This case is the flip side of Ethics Mini-Case 1. Here, a lower price (and copayment) is quoted to the patient while the insurer pays a higher amount.

Mini-Case 4: This case focuses on the personal conflicts that arise when the CEO of a small, not-for-profit hospital is confronted with multiple takeover bids.

Mini-Case 5: This case discusses the dilemma that hospitals face in treating the uninsured. How much should hospitals charge the uninsured for services provided, and how aggressively should they pursue those collections?

Mini-Case 6: This case centers on the financial arrangements being used by some imaging services companies to "encourage" physicians to refer patients to their centers. Are these arrangements legal? If so, are the arrangements ethical?

Mini-Case 7: This case focuses on physician-owned distributorships, whereby physicians (primarily orthopedic surgeons) have an ownership interest in the companies that furnish the medical devices used in their surgical procedures. Do these companies raise any legal or ethical issues?

Financial
Accounting

RIVER COMMUNITY HOSPITAL (A)

ASSESSING HOSPITAL PERFORMANCE

1

RIVER COMMUNITY HOSPITAL is a 210-bed, not-for-profit, acute care hospital with a long-standing reputation for providing quality healthcare services to a growing service area. River competes with three other hospitals in its metropolitan statistical area (MSA)—two not-for-profit and one for-profit. It is the smallest of the four but has traditionally been ranked highest in patient satisfaction polls.

Hospitals are accredited by The Joint Commission, an independent, not-for-profit organization whose mission is to improve the safety and quality of healthcare provided to the public through accreditation and related services. (For more information on The Joint Commission, visit its website at www.jointcommission.org.) Although accreditation is optional for hospitals, it is generally required to qualify for governmental (Medicare and Medicaid) reimbursement, and hence the vast majority of hospitals apply for accreditation. River passed its latest Joint Commission survey with "flying colors," receiving the Gold Seal of Approval from that accrediting body.

In recent years, competition among the four hospitals in River's service area has been keen but friendly. However, a large for-profit chain recently purchased the for-profit hospital, which has resulted in some anxiety among the managers of the other three hospitals because of the chain's reputation for aggressively increasing market share in the markets they serve.

Relevant financial and operating data for River are contained in Exhibits 1.1 through 1.5, and selected industry data are contained in

Exhibits 1.6 and 1.7. (Note that the industry data given in the case are for illustrative purposes only and do not represent actual data for the years specified. For a better idea of the type of comparative data actually available for hospitals, see the Optum™ website at www.hospital benchmarks.com.)

In addition to the data in the exhibits, the following information was extracted from the notes section of River's 2013 Annual Report.

1. A significant portion of the hospital's net patient service revenue was generated by patients who are covered either by Medicare, Medicaid, or other government programs or by various private plans, including managed care plans, that have contracts with the hospital that specify discounts from charges. In general, the proportional amount of deductions is similar between inpatients and outpatients. The gross and net patient service revenue and operating expenses breakdown for both inpatient and outpatient services is given in Exhibit 1.4.

2. River has a contributory money accumulation (defined contribution) pension plan that covers substantially all of its employees. Participants can contribute up to 20 percent of earnings to the pension plan. The hospital matches, on a dollar-for-dollar basis, employee contributions of up to 2 percent of wages and pays 50 cents on the dollar for contributions over 2 percent and up to 4 percent. Because the plan is a defined contribution plan (as opposed to a defined benefit plan), River has no unfunded pension liabilities. Pension expense was approximately $0.543 million in 2012 and $0.588 million in 2013.

3. The hospital is a member of the State Hospital Trust Fund, under which it purchases professional liability insurance coverage for individual claims up to $1 million (subject to a deductible of $100,000 per claim). River is self-insured for amounts above $1 million but less than $5 million. Any liability award in excess of $5 million is covered by a commercial liability policy; for example, the policy pays $2 million on a $7 million award. The hospital is currently involved

in eight suits involving claims of various amounts that could ultimately be tried before juries. Although it is impossible to determine the exact potential liability in these claims, management does not believe that the settlement of these cases would have a material effect on the hospital's financial position.

Assume that you have just joined the staff of River Community Hospital as a special assistant to the CEO. On your first day on the job, the CEO, Melissa Randolph, stated that the best way to get to know the financial and operating condition of the hospital is to conduct a thorough financial statement and operating indicator analysis; thus, she assigned you the task. Although you also believe that this is a good way to get started, you wonder whether Melissa has any ulterior motives. Perhaps the hospital is having problems and she thinks that you can spot them, or perhaps she wants to test your analytical skills. Melissa is from the "old school" of hospital management and has been looking for someone to bring modern management methods to the hospital.

As you prepare for the presentation, several relevant factors come to light. First, in reviewing the policy decisions made by River's board of trustees over the past decade, you note that in 2008 the board made the decision to significantly expand the hospital's outpatient services. The rationale was that many procedures that historically were done on an inpatient basis were now being done in an outpatient setting, and if River did not offer such services it would lose the patients to other providers.

Second, the board chair has great concern about the decline in profitability between 2011 and 2012 and has not been assuaged by the recent modest upturn. Perhaps because she is CEO of a local company, the chair focuses on return on equity (ROE) as the key measure of profitability. She has requested that management develop some strategies to improve profitability and estimate the impact of the strategies on the hospital's ROE.

Third, you discover that board members were complaining that too much time is being spent at quarterly board meetings discussing the hospital's financial condition. "There is so much to accomplish," said one member, "that we just don't have the time to consider a large number of ratios at each meeting."

You know that many healthcare providers are now using dashboards to focus on key performance indicators (KPIs). A dashboard is nothing more than a way to summarize an organization's financial and operating performance. Of course, the name stems from an automobile's dashboard, which contains gauges that give drivers essential information about the car's performance and operating condition. Thus, you plan to develop two dashboards, each containing no more than five KPIs. One dashboard will use financial ratios to focus on financial performance, while the other will use operating indicator ratios to focus on operating performance. You plan to present your recommendations for the contents of these dashboards, along with the rationale for the ratios chosen, at the board meeting. Your ultimate goal is to replace the full financial and operating performance discussion at future board meetings with a limited discussion of the KPIs.

EXHIBIT 1.1	2011	2012	2013
River Community Hospital: Statements of Operations (millions of dollars)			
Revenues			
Net patient service revenue	$28.796	$30.576	$34.582
Other revenue	1.237	1.853	1.834
Total revenues	$30.033	$32.429	$36.416
Expenses			
Salaries and wages	$12.245	$12.468	$13.994
Fringe benefits	1.830	2.408	2.568
Interest expense	1.181	1.598	1.776
Depreciation	2.350	2.658	2.778
Medical supplies and drugs	0.622	0.655	0.776
Professional liability	0.140	0.201	0.218
Other	9.036	10.339	11.848
Total expenses	$27.404	$30.327	$33.958
Net Income	$ 2.629	$ 2.102	$ 2.458

	2011	2012	2013
Assets			
Cash and investments	$ 4.673	$ 5.069	$ 2.795
Accounts receivable (net)	4.359	5.674	7.413
Inventories	0.432	0.523	0.601
Other current assets	0.308	0.703	0.923
Total current assets	$ 9.772	$11.969	$11.732
Gross plant and equipment	$47.786	$55.333	$59.552
Accumulated depreciation	11.820	14.338	17.009
Net plant and equipment	$35.966	$40.995	$42.543
Total assets	$45.738	$52.964	$54.275
Liabilities and Net Assets			
Accounts payable	$ 0.928	$ 1.253	$ 1.760
Accrued expenses	1.460	1.503	1.176
Current portion of LT debt	0.110	1.341	1.465
Total current liabilities	$ 2.498	$ 4.097	$ 4.401
Long-term debt	15.673	19.222	17.795
Net assets	27.567	29.645	32.079
Total liabilities and net assets	$45.738	$52.964	$54.275

LT: long term

EXHIBIT 1.2
River Community Hospital: Balance Sheets (millions of dollars)

EXHIBIT 1.3
River Community
Hospital: Statements of
Cash Flows
(millions of dollars)

	2012	2013
Cash Flows from Operating Activities		
Net income	$2.102	$2.458
Depreciation and noncash expenses	2.633	2.756
Change in accounts receivable	(1.315)	(1.739)
Change in inventories	(0.091)	(0.078)
Change in other current assets	(0.395)	(0.220)
Change in accounts payable	0.325	0.507
Change in accrued expenses	0.043	(0.327)
Net cash flow from operations	$3.302	$3.357
Cash Flows from Investing Activities		
Investment in plant and equipment	($7.686)	($4.328)
Cash Flows from Financing Activities		
Change in long-term debt	$3.549	($1.427)
Change in current portion		
of long-term debt	$1.231	$0.124
Net cash flow from financing	$4.780	($1.303)
Net increase (decrease) in cash	$0.396	($2.274)
Beginning cash	$4.673	$5.069
Ending cash	$5.069	$2.795

Note: "Depreciation and noncash expenses" and "Investment in plant and equipment" data in the statements of cash flows are somewhat different than they would be if calculated directly from the other financial statements because of asset revaluations.

	2011	2012	2013
Operating Revenue			
Gross inpatient service	$26.117	$29.148	$33.216
Gross outpatient service	6.535	9.130	11.912
Gross patient service revenue	$32.652	$38.278	$45.128
Contractual allowances	$ 1.729	$ 5.196	$ 7.516
Bad debt and charity care	2.127	2.506	3.030
Total revenue deductions	$ 3.856	$7.702	$10.546
Net patient service revenue	$28.796	$30.576	$34.582
Operating Expenses			
Inpatient service	$20.573	$22.229	$24.771
Outpatient service	6.831	8.098	9.187
Total operating expenses	$27.404	$30.327	$33.958

EXHIBIT 1.4
River Community Hospital: Revenue and Expense Allocation (millions of dollars)

	2011	2012	2013
Medicare discharges	2,721	2,860	2,741
Total discharges	8,784	8,318	8,576
Outpatient visits	32,285	32,878	36,796
Licensed beds	210	210	210
Staffed beds	193	197	178
Patient days	44,085	42,434	40,062
All-payer case mix index	1.2869	1.2993	1.3161
Full-time equivalents	610.8	625.8	619.3

EXHIBIT 1.5
River Community Hospital: Selected Operating Data

EXHIBIT 1.6
2013 Selected Industry
Financial Ratios
(200–299 beds)

	+Quartile	Median	−Quartile
Profitability Ratios			
Total margin	5.58%	3.48%	0.53%
Return on assets	5.80%	3.10%	0.40%
Return on equity	15.66%	6.01%	0.62%
Deductible ratio[a]	0.34	0.26	0.18
Liquidity Ratios			
Current ratio	2.53	1.99	1.48
Days cash on hand	32.35	15.89	6.24
Debt Management Ratios			
Debt ratio	62.90%	48.40%	35.20%
Debt to equity ratio	127.00%	64.70%	26.90%
Times interest earned	4.29	2.23	1.14
Cash flow coverage	5.32	3.22	1.76
Asset Management Ratios			
Fixed asset turnover	2.20	1.76	1.49
Total asset turnover	1.04	0.89	0.75
Days in patient accounts receivable	87.53	75.67	63.33
Current asset turnover[b]	3.94	3.38	2.88
Average payment period (days)[c]	71.24	56.52	45.84
Other Ratios			
Average age of plant (years)	8.86	7.39	6.14

[a]Deductions/Gross patient service revenue
[b]Total revenues/Current assets
[c]Current liabilities/[(Total expenses − Depreciation expense)/365]

Notes: 1. The industry data shown here are for illustrative purposes only and hence should not be used outside this case.

2. The upper quartile is based on the higher numerical value for the ratio and the lower quartile on the lower numerical value, regardless of whether a high value is good or bad. The interpretation is left to the analyst.

	+Quartile	Median	−Quartile
Profit Indicators			
Profit per discharge[a]	$89.04	($21.30)	($120.08)
Profit per visit[b]	$ 6.22	$ 0.66	($ 7.01)
Net Revenue Indicators			
Net revenue per discharge[c]	$4,091	$3,411	$2,815
Net revenue per visit[d]	$ 201	$ 139	$ 98
Medicare revenue percentage[e]	43.47%	36.60%	31.25%
Bad debt/charity care percentage[f]	7.89%	4.76%	2.97%
Contractual allowance percentage[g]	25.27%	20.02%	12.12%
Outpatient revenue percentage[h]	25.26%	21.03%	17.44%
Volume Indicators			
Occupancy rate[i]	67.12%	58.10%	47.84%
Average daily census[j]	173.23	144.73	114.39
Length-of-Stay Indicators			
Average length of stay (days)[k]	6.80	6.07	5.41
Adjusted length of stay[l]	6.48	5.36	4.52
Intensity-of-Service Indicators			
Expense per discharge[m]	$ 3,937	$ 3,392	$ 2,972
Adjusted expense per discharge[n]	$ 3,417	$ 2,924	$ 2,572
Expense per visit[o]	$202.23	$141.97	$111.53
All-payer case mix index[p]	1.2795	1.1756	1.0259
Efficiency Indicators			
FTEs per occupied bed[q]	4.59	4.15	3.77
Labor-hours per visit[r]	4.68	5.84	8.66
Unit Cost Indicators			
Salary per FTE[s]	$24,447	$22,517	$20,347
Employee benefits percentage[t]	19.58%	17.04%	15.18%
Liability expense per discharge[u]	$ 80.94	$ 42.05	$ 18.31

EXHIBIT 1.7
2013 Selected Industry Operating Ratios (200–299 beds)

[a](Net inpatient revenue − Inpatient expenses)/Total discharges
[b](Net outpatient revenue − Outpatient expenses)/Total visits
[c]Net inpatient revenue/Total discharges

^{d}Net outpatient revenue/Total visits

^{e}Medicare net patient revenue/Total net patient revenue

^{f}(Bad debt + Charity care)/Gross patient revenue

^{g}Contractual allowances/Gross patient revenue

^{h}Net outpatient revenue/Total net patient revenue

^{i}Patient days/(Staffed beds × 365)

^{j}Patient days/365

^{k}Patient days/Total discharges

^{l}Average length of stay/Case mix index

^{m}Inpatient expenses/Total discharges

^{n}Expense per discharge/Case mix index

^{o}Outpatient expenses/Total visits

^{p}Sum of DRG weights/Total discharges

^{q}Inpatient FTEs/Average daily census

^{r}(Outpatient FTEs × 2,080)/Total visits

^{s}Total salaries/Total FTEs

^{t}Fringe benefit expense/Total salaries

^{u}Inpatient professional liability expense/Total discharges

DRG: diagnosis-related group; FTE: full-time equivalent

Notes: 1. The industry data shown here are for illustrative purposes only and hence should not be used outside this case.

2. The upper quartile is based on the higher numerical value for the ratio and the lower quartile on the lower numerical value, regardless of whether a high value is good or bad. The interpretation is left to the analyst.

COMMONWEALTH HEALTH PLANS

ASSESSING HMO PERFORMANCE

2

COMMONWEALTH HEALTH PLANS is one of Virginia's largest managed care organizations (MCOs). In fact, it is the largest of the state's not-for-profit MCOs. It offers prepaid health coverage to more than 500,000 members in 17 counties, including the following major cities: Richmond, Norfolk, Virginia Beach, Arlington, Alexandria, and Roanoke.

Commonwealth's various products include commercial health maintenance organizations (HMOs), Medicare HMOs (Medicare Advantage plans), preferred provider organizations (PPOs), and point-of-service (POS) plans. These plans are all designed to meet the needs of a wide segment of Virginia's population of approximately 8 million. The revenue breakdown of plan types is as follows:

Plan Type	Percent of Revenue
Commercial HMO	46
Medicare HMO	39
PPO	10
POS	5
	100

Commonwealth was the first managed care organization in Virginia to seek and receive accreditation from the National Committee for Quality Assurance (NCQA), and each of its component plans has been rated as excellent, the highest accreditation level. The NCQA judges a

13

health plan on its performance in three areas: clinical performance (based on HEDIS [Healthcare Effectiveness Data and Information Set] results), member satisfaction (based on CAHPS [Consumer Assessment of Healthcare Providers and Systems] results), and a review of key structures and processes. HEDIS and CAHPS scores together account for about 40 percent of the assessment for HMOs, with performance against structure and process standards accounting for the remaining 60 percent. All three areas are important, and together they give an accurate overall assessment of the quality of a health plan. (For more information on the NCQA, visit its website at www.ncqa.org.)

A summary of Commonwealth's 2012 and 2013 HMO plan financial data (including both commercial and Medicare) is presented in Exhibit 2.1, while Exhibit 2.2 contains a summary of operating and enrollment data. To help in analyzing Commonwealth's performance, its managers have classified the following four Virginia HMOs as "primary competitors."

HMO	Number of Counties Served	2013 Total Enrollment	2013 Total Assets (000s)
WellLife	23	516,858	$408,707
Signet Healthcare	15	360,252	178,662
Proxima	15	247,109	144,982
Sparta	28	205,296	103,504

These plans have the geographic coverage and financial resources to be prominent players in the Virginia managed care industry. Furthermore, the primary competitors are operating in the same service areas and have a similar product mix as Commonwealth and hence are potential threats to its future success. In addition to comparisons with national data, all internal analyses that use benchmarking compare Commonwealth's performance with the state average as well as with the primary competitor list. **Note, however, that not all relevant performance measures have a complete set of comparative data available.**

Exhibit 2.3 contains selected financial and operating ratios for Commonwealth's primary competitors as well as the means and medians for all Virginia HMOs. Exhibit 2.4 contains selected national data, in which all comparative data are for HMO plans only. Exhibit 2.5 contains selected ratio definitions. (For a better understanding of the types of comparative data available for managed care plans, see the HealthLeaders-InterStudy website at www.hl-isy.com.)

Assume that you have just started an administrative residency at Commonwealth Health Plans. On your first day at the organization, Robert Osborne, the chief executive officer, stated that the best way to get to know the financial and operating condition of any business is to do a brief financial statement and operating indicator analysis; thus, he assigned you the task. Although you agree that this is a great way to learn more about Commonwealth and its competitors' HMO plans, you wonder whether he has any hidden motives. Perhaps the company is having financial problems with these plans and he thinks that you can spot them, or perhaps he just wants to test your analytical skills.

In any event, he has already scheduled a financial and operating performance analysis presentation for the next executive committee meeting as a way for you to demonstrate your skills to Commonwealth's senior managers. In preparing for the meeting, you called Amity Wallace, the previous administrative resident, to get some hints on how to prepare for your presentation to the executive committee. Amity just left Commonwealth for a great job with Humana. Her advice was to do a standard financial statement analysis, including statement of cash flows analysis, Du Pont analysis, and ratio and operating indicator analyses.

Your first impression was that this task should be a "piece of cake," as you had performed a similar analysis for a hospital during your internship. However, as you began the task, it became apparent that the ratios used and their interpretations differ across industries; that is, the ratios that are critical to identifying the financial condition of a hospital are not necessarily the same ratios that are critical to a managed care plan. In addition, many of the ratios that are relevant to both hospitals and managed care plans have values that differ substantially.

To illustrate, consider the medical loss ratio (defined as medical expenses divided by premium revenue), which measures the proportion of premium revenue that is spent on providing member healthcare services. Clearly, this ratio is not applicable to providers such as hospitals. Interestingly, healthcare reform (the Affordable Care Act) mandates that large group insurance plans spend at least 85 percent of premiums on medical services. If they fail to meet this requirement, insurers must pay a rebate to customers. (Does Commonwealth meet this requirement? Also, what do think of the choice of terminology for the medical loss ratio?)

To help the executive committee interpret your presentation, you plan to point out key differences between your analysis for a health plan and that for a hospital as they emerge. In addition, you know that it is more important to identify key areas of concern and to recommend courses of action than it is to merely go over the numbers.

	2012	2013
Statements of Operations		
Premium revenue	$313.7	$357.6
Interest income	2.4	3.5
Total revenues	$316.1	$361.1
Operating expenses:		
Medical costs	$263.0	$291.8
Selling and administrative	36.8	43.6
Depreciation	4.7	5.0
Total operating expenses	$304.5	$340.4
Net income	$ 11.6	$ 20.7
Balance Sheets		
Cash	$ 37.2	$ 27.2
Marketable securities	42.7	60.9
Premiums receivable	3.7	7.4
Total current assets	$ 83.6	$ 95.5
Net fixed assets	30.0	31.7
Total assets	$113.6	$127.2
Medical costs payable	$ 44.8	$ 48.7
Accounts payable/accruals	15.4	17.3
Total current liabilities	$ 60.2	$ 66.0
Long-term debt	17.1	4.2
Net assets (equity)	36.3	57.0
Total liabilities and net assets	$113.6	$127.2
Other Data		
Medical loss ratio	83.8%	81.6%
Administrative cost ratio	13.2%	13.6%
Total commercial premium revenue	$170.9	$205.6
Total Medicare revenue	$142.8	$152.0
Total physician services expense	$125.6	$127.1
Total inpatient expense	$ 80.8	$ 90.1
Total other medical expense	$ 56.6	$ 74.6

EXHIBIT 2.1
Commonwealth Health Plans: HMO Plan Financial Data (millions of dollars)

EXHIBIT 2.2
Commonwealth Health Plans: HMO Plan Operating and Enrollment Data (millions of dollars)

	2012	2013
Commercial premium revenue PMPM	$127.82	$127.90
Medicare revenue PMPM	$449.37	$437.23
Commercial patient days per 1,000 enrollees	302.9	266.4
Medicare patient days per 1,000 enrollees	1,622.4	1,418.1
Commercial member-months	1,337,036	1,607,036
Commercial physician encounters	594,381	622,749
Commercial inpatient days	43,661	39,763
Medicare member-months	317,778	347,643
Medicare physician encounters	149,622	185,283

PMPM: per member per month

EXHIBIT 2.3
Selected State HMO Industry Financial and Operating Data (millions of dollars)

	2012	2013
Total Margin		
WellLife	4.8%	5.8%
Signet Healthcare	3.0	3.2
Proxima	9.1	(0.7)
Sparta	10.5	9.1
State average	3.8	(3.9)
State median	4.8	4.7
Percent Administrative Expense		
WellLife	12.1%	11.5%
Signet Healthcare	12.2	13.4
Proxima	13.6	16.4
Sparta	23.9	26.8
State average	15.5	17.4
State median	14.8	15.7
Percent Inpatient Expense		
WellLife	32.2%	30.3%
Signet Healthcare	22.8	22.4
Proxima	21.2	23.0
Sparta	18.2	18.8
State average	25.2	23.3
State median	23.6	24.3

	2012	2013
Percent Physician Expense		
WellLife	54.1%	56.9%
Signet Healthcare	31.3	30.3
Proxima	22.7	24.9
Sparta	12.8	18.6
State average	28.8	31.3
State median	31.1	31.6
Percent Other Medical Expense		
WellLife	0.1%	0.1%
Signet Healthcare	8.9	7.8
Proxima	27.5	30.2
Sparta	45.7	35.0
State average	14.6	12.5
State median	10.2	8.9
Commercial Premium Revenue PMPM		
WellLife	$108.68	$110.19
Signet Healthcare	39.86	27.50
Proxima	120.68	124.27
Sparta	88.41	95.06
State average	101.17	102.53
State median	108.32	108.95
Medicare Revenue PMPM		
WellLife	$406.57	$421.57
Signet Healthcare	N/A	N/A
Proxima	N/A	N/A
Sparta	N/A	N/A
State average	365.12	376.04
State median	426.18	430.57
Commercial Inpatient Days per 1,000 Enrollees		
WellLife	245.4	246.0
Signet Healthcare	258.4	248.8
Proxima	251.8	259.2
Sparta	198.2	248.9
State average	278.0	237.0
State median	279.1	248.8

EXHIBIT 2.3 (continued) Selected State HMO Industry Financial and Operating Data (millions of dollars)

EXHIBIT 2.3
(continued)
Selected State HMO
Industry Financial and
Operating Data
(millions of dollars)

	2012	*2013*
Medicare Inpatient Days per 1,000 Enrollees		
WellLife	1,388.4	1,323.8
Signet Healthcare	1,165.2	1,188.7
Proxima	1,518.8	1,382.2
Sparta	1,623.8	1,566.9
State average	1,432.1	1,375.5
State median	1,380.5	1,350.6
Commercial Physician Encounters per Member		
WellLife	2.2	3.6
Signet Healthcare	1.5	1.4
Proxima	2.7	2.6
Sparta	3.5	3.6
State average	3.8	3.8
State median	3.9	3.7
Medicare Physician Encounters per Member		
WellLife	9.8	9.6
Signet Healthcare	6.6	6.9
Proxima	10.1	10.0
Sparta	11.2	11.3
State average	9.1	9.1
State median	8.6	8.9

Note: The Virginia data for the HMO industry contained in this exhibit are for illustrative purposes only. These data should not be used to conduct actual financial analyses.

Average copay per office visit	$ 8	
Average copay per hospitalization	$36	
Average copay per pharmacy prescription	$ 7	
Medical Loss Ratio		
Upper quartile	89.0%	
Median	84.9	
Lower quartile	80.0	
Administrative Cost Ratio		
Upper quartile	14.4%	
Median	12.0	
Lower quartile	9.0	
Operating Margin		
Upper quartile	5.0%	
Median	2.5	
Lower quartile	1.1	
Total Margin		
Upper quartile	5.5%	
Median	2.9	
Lower quartile	1.5	
Return on Assets (ROA)		
Upper quartile	16.5%	
Median	11.3	
Lower quartile	4.8	
Return on Equity (ROE)		
Upper quartile	50.2%	
Median	31.4	
Lower quartile	18.2	
Current Ratio		
Upper quartile	1.29	
Median	0.95	
Lower quartile	0.49	
Days Cash on Hand		
Upper quartile	32.7	
Median	10.3	
Lower quartile	0.8	

EXHIBIT 2.4
Selected 2013 National HMO Industry Financial and Operating Data

**EXHIBIT 2.4
(continued)
Selected 2013 National
HMO Industry Financial
and Operating Data**

Current Asset Turnover

Upper quartile	14.1
Median	6.4
Lower quartile	3.7

Total Asset Turnover

Upper quartile	4.1
Median	3.1
Lower quartile	2.2

Days Premiums Receivable

Upper quartile	14.0
Median	8.9
Lower quartile	7.0

Debt Ratio

Upper quartile	81.3%
Median	68.4
Lower quartile	59.7

Note: The national data for the HMO industry contained in this exhibit are for illustrative purposes only. These data should not be used to conduct actual financial analyses.

**EXHIBIT 2.5
Selected Ratio
Definitions**

Medical Loss Ratio

$$\frac{\text{Medical expenses}}{\text{Premium revenue}}$$

Administrative Cost Ratio

$$\frac{\text{Selling and administrative expenses} + \text{Depreciation}}{\text{Premium revenue}}$$

Operating Margin

$$\frac{\text{Net income} - \text{Interest income}}{\text{Premium revenue}}$$

Percent Administrative Expense

$$\frac{\text{Selling and administrative expense}}{\text{Total operating expenses}}$$

Percent Inpatient Expense

$$\frac{\text{Inpatient expense}}{\text{Total operating expenses}}$$

Percent Physician Expense

$$\frac{\text{Physician services expense}}{\text{Total operating expenses}}$$

Percent Other Medical Expense

$$\frac{\text{Other medical expense}}{\text{Total operating expenses}}$$

Managerial
Accounting

BIG BEND MEDICAL CENTER

3

COST ALLOCATION
CONCEPTS

Big Bend Medical Center is a full-service, not-for-profit, acute care hospital with 325 beds located in Big Bend, Texas. The bulk of the hospital's facilities are devoted to inpatient care and emergency services. However, a 100,000-square-foot section of the hospital complex is devoted to outpatient services. Currently, this space has two primary uses. About 80 percent of the space is used by the Outpatient Clinic, which handles all routine outpatient services offered by the hospital. The remaining 20 percent is used by the Dialysis Center.

The Dialysis Center performs hemodialysis and peritoneal dialysis, which are alternative processes that remove wastes and excess water from the blood for patients with end-stage renal (kidney) disease. In hemodialysis, blood is pumped from the patient's arm through a shunt into a dialysis machine, which uses a cleansing solution and an artificial membrane to perform the functions of a healthy kidney. Then, the cleansed blood is pumped back into the patient through a second shunt.

In peritoneal dialysis, the cleansing solution is inserted directly into the abdominal cavity through a catheter. The body naturally cleanses the blood through the peritoneum—a thin membrane that lines the abdominal cavity.

Typically, hemodialysis patients require three dialyses a week, with each treatment lasting about four hours. Patients who use peritoneal dialysis change their own cleansing solutions at home, usually about six times per day. This procedure can be done manually when active or automatically by machine when sleeping. However, the patient's overall condition, as well as the positioning of the catheter, must be monitored regularly by nurses and technicians at the Dialysis Center.

Big Bend's cost accounting system, which was installed two years ago, allocates facilities costs (which at Big Bend essentially consist of building depreciation and interest on long-term debt) on the basis of square footage. Currently, the facilities cost allocation rate is $15 per square foot, so the facilities cost allocation is $20,000 \times \$15 = \$300,000$ for the Dialysis Center and $80,000 \times \$15 = \$1,200,000$ for the Outpatient Clinic. All other overhead costs, such as administration, finance, maintenance, and housekeeping, are lumped together and called "general overhead." These costs are allocated on the basis of 10 percent of the revenues of each patient service department. The current allocation of general overhead is $270,000 for the Dialysis Center and $1,600,000 for the Outpatient Clinic, which results in total overhead allocations of $570,000 for the Dialysis Center and $2,800,000 for the Outpatient Clinic.

Recent growth in volume of the Outpatient Clinic has created a need for 25 percent more space than is currently assigned. Because the Outpatient Clinic is much larger than the Dialysis Center, and because the Clinic's patients need frequent access to other departments within the hospital, the decision was made to keep the Outpatient Clinic in its current location and to move the Dialysis Center to another location to free up space within the hospital complex. Such a move would boost the Outpatient Clinic space to 100,000 square feet, a 25 percent increase.

After attempting to find space for the Dialysis Center within the hospital complex, it was soon determined that a new 20,000-square-foot building must be built. This building would be situated three blocks away from the hospital complex, in a location that would be much more convenient for dialysis patients (and Center employees) because of ease of parking. The 20,000 square feet of space, which can be more efficiently used than the old space, allows for some increase in patient volume, although it is unclear whether or not the move will generate additional dialysis patients.

Construction cost of the new building is estimated at $120 per square foot, for a total cost of $2,400,000. Additionally, the purchase of land, furniture, and other fittings, along with the relocation of equipment, files, and other items, would cost $1,600,000, for a total cost of $4,000,000. The $4,000,000 cost would be financed by a 7.75 percent, 20-year, first-mortgage loan. When both the principal amount (which can be considered depreciation) and interest are amortized over 20 years, the end result is an annual cost of financing of $400,000. Thus, it is possible to estimate the actual annual facilities costs for the new Dialysis Center, something that is not possible for units located within the hospital complex.

Exhibit 3.1 contains the projected profit and loss (P&L) statement for the Dialysis Center before adjusting for the move. Big Bend's department heads receive annual bonuses on the basis of each department's contribution to the hospital's bottom line (profit). In the past, only direct costs were considered, but Big Bend's CEO has decided that bonuses will now be based on full (total) costs.

The new approach to awarding bonuses, coupled with the potential increases in indirect cost allocation, is of great concern to John Van Pelt, the director of the Dialysis Center. Under the current allocation of indirect costs (see Exhibit 3.1), John would have a reasonable chance of earning an end-of-year bonus, as the forecast puts the Dialysis Center in the black. However, any increase in the indirect cost allocation would likely put him out of the money.

At the next department heads' meeting, John voiced his concern about the impact of any allocation changes on the Dialysis Center's reported profitability, so Big Bend's CEO asked the chief financial officer (CFO), Rick Simmons, to look into the matter. In essence, the CEO said that the final allocation is up to Rick but that any allocation changes must be made within outpatient services. In other words, any change in indirect cost allocation to the Dialysis Center must be offset by an equal, but opposite, change in the allocation to the Outpatient Clinic.

To get started, Rick created Exhibit 3.2. In creating the exhibit, Rick assumed that the new Dialysis Center would have the same number of stations as the old one, would serve the same number of patients, and would receive the same reimbursement rates. Also, direct operating expenses would differ only slightly from the current situation because the same personnel and equipment would be used. Thus, for all practical purposes, the revenues and direct costs of the Dialysis Center would be unaffected by the move.

The data in Exhibit 3.2 for the expanded Outpatient Clinic are based on the assumption that the expansion would allow volume to increase by 25 percent and that both revenues and direct costs would increase by a like amount. Furthermore, to keep the analysis manageable, the assumption was made that the overall hospital allocation rates for both facilities costs and general overhead would not materially change as a result of the expansion.

Rick knew that his "trial balloon" allocation, which is shown in Exhibit 3.2 in the columns labeled "Initial Allocation," would create some controversy. In the past, facilities costs were aggregated, so all departments were charged a cost based on the average embedded (historical) cost regardless of the actual age (or value) of the space occupied. Thus, a basement room with no windows was allocated the same facilities costs (per square foot) as was the fifth floor executive suite. Because many department heads considered this approach to be unfair, Rick wanted to begin allocating facilities overhead on a true cost basis. Thus, in his initial allocation, Rick used actual facilities costs as the basis for the allocation to the Dialysis Center.

Needless to say, John's response to the initial allocation was less than enthusiastic. Specifically, he was concerned over several issues. First and foremost, is it fair for the Dialysis Center to suffer (in terms of profitability) because it will be charged actual facilities costs for its new location? After all, the move was forced by the Outpatient Clinic, which is being charged for facilities at the lower average allocation rate. Under the concept of charging for actual facilities costs, department heads might be better off by resisting proposed moves to new (and potentially more efficient) facilities because such moves would result in increased facilities allocations.

Also, even if the actual cost concept were applied to the Dialysis Center, is the $400,000 annual allocation amount correct? After all, the building has a useful life that is probably significantly longer than 20 years—the life of the loan used to determine the allocation amount. If the true cost concept is applied, what would be the allocation in the 21st year, after the mortgage had been paid off?

Finally, it appears that the revenue the Dialysis Center "receives" from patient use of the pharmacy is passed on directly to the pharmacy. That is, the Dialysis Center books $800,000 in annual revenue but then is charged $800,000 for the drugs used. Should this "revenue" be counted when general overhead allocations are made? To make his point, John discovered that the pharmacy supplies used for dialysis actually cost the pharmacy $400,000, so the pharmacy makes a profit of $400,000 on drugs that are actually "sold" by the Dialysis Center.

Before Rick was able to respond to John's concerns, he suddenly left Big Bend to be the CFO of a competing investor-owned hospital. The task of completing the allocation study was given to you, Big Bend's current administrative resident. You remember that to be of most benefit to the organization, cost allocations should (1) be perceived as fair by the parties involved and (2) promote overall cost savings within the organization. However, you also realize that, in practice, cost allocation is very complex and somewhat arbitrary. Some department heads argue that the best approach to overhead allocations is the "Marxist approach," by which allocations are based on each patient service department's ability to cover overhead costs.

Considering all the relevant issues, you must develop and justify a new indirect cost allocation scheme for outpatient services. Summarize your results in the "Alternative Allocation" columns in Exhibit 3.2, and be prepared to justify your recommendations at the next department heads' meeting.

Revenues		
Hemodialysis program		$1,300,000
Peritoneal dialysis program		600,000
Pharmaceutical supplies		800,000
Total revenues		$2,700,000
Direct Expenses		
Salaries and benefits		$ 900,000
Pharmaceutical supplies		800,000
Other medical/administrative supplies		100,000
Utilities		80,000
Equipment lease expense		120,000
Other expenses		100,000
Total expenses		$2,100,000
Net gain (loss) before indirect costs		$ 600,000
Indirect Expenses		
Facilities costs		$ 300,000
General overhead		270,000
Total overhead costs		$ 570,000
Net profit		$ 30,000

EXHIBIT 3.1
Big Bend Medical Center
Dialysis Center: Pro
Forma P&L Statement
Assuming Status Quo

Note: Pharmacy revenues are based on reimbursement amounts, not costs.

EXHIBIT 3.2
Big Bend Medical Center: Dialysis Center (DC) and Outpatient Clinic (OC) Summary Projections

P&L Statements:

| | Without Expansion | | With Expansion | | | |
| | | | Initial Allocation | | Alternative Allocation | |
	DC	OC	DC	OC	DC	OC
Revenues/Direct Costs						
Total revenues	$ 2,700,000	$16,000,000	$ 2,700,000	$20,000,000	$ 2,700,000	$20,000,000
Direct expenses	2,100,000	9,833,155	2,100,000	12,291,444	2,100,000	12,291,444
Contribution margin	$ 600,000	$ 6,166,845	$ 600,000	$ 7,708,556	$ 600,000	$ 7,708,556
Percent of revenues	22.2%	38.5%	22.2%	38.5%	22.2%	38.5%
Indirect Costs						
Facilities costs	$ 300,000	$ 1,200,000	$ 400,000	$ 1,500,000	$	$
General overhead	270,000	1,600,000	270,000	2,000,000		
Total overhead	$ 570,000	$ 2,800,000	$ 670,000	$ 3,500,000	$	$
Net profit	$ 30,000	$ 3,366,845	($ 70,000)	$ 4,208,556	$	$
Percent of revenues	1.1%	21.0%	(2.6%)	21.0%	%	%
Facilities Cost Allocation:						
Square footage	20,000	80,000	20,000	100,000	20,000	100,000
Facilities costs per square foot	$ 15.00	$ 15.00	$ 20.00	$ 15.00	$	$
Other Overhead Allocation:						
General overhead costs as a % of revenue	10.0%	10.0%	10.0%	10.0%	%	%

Note: The term "contribution margin" as used here means the amount available to cover overhead costs, as opposed to the traditional meaning of the amount available to cover fixed costs.

EAGAN FAMILY PRACTICE

COST ALLOCATION
METHODS

4

EAGAN FAMILY PRACTICE (the Group) is a medical practice with four locations in the Minneapolis/St. Paul area. The clinical staff consists of 20 physicians—all of whom practice in one or more areas of family medicine—and 46 physician extenders and nurses. The Group is organized into three patient services departments: Adult Medicine, Obstetrics, and Pediatrics. Supporting these patient service departments are three support departments: Administration, Facilities, and Finance. Exhibit 4.1 contains the Group's summary revenue and cost projections by department for the coming year.

As part of a much-needed overhaul of the cost allocation process, the Group contracted with a major accounting firm to estimate the amount of services provided by the support departments to each other and to each patient service department. The intent of the study was to provide data that would help the Group develop a better cost allocation system to replace the outdated, arbitrary system currently in use. The results of this study are shown in Exhibit 4.2. Although expressed as percentages of the total dollar amount of support provided to other departments (instead of the more typical cost allocation rates), the data in Exhibit 4.2 are based on an extensive study using sound managerial accounting techniques. Thus, both senior management and department heads at the Group are comfortable with the resulting allocation percentages. **(Hint: To ensure that you apply the percentages properly in your analysis, pay attention to Note 2 at the bottom of Exhibit 4.2.)**

The second step in the cost allocation process improvement initiative is to choose the allocation method. There are four allocation methods under consideration: direct, step-down, double apportionment, and reciprocal. To aid in the decision, Jerry Silverman, the Group's finance chief, has asked Ashley Matson, an administrative resident at the Group, to conduct a study and to make a recommendation regarding the best allocation method.

There are several possible approaches to the task, but Ashley has decided to "examine by doing." That is, she plans to use the data in Exhibits 4.1 and 4.2 to determine the overhead cost allocations under each method. Once this is done, she will be able to compare and contrast the results.

Of course, the final decision cannot be made without considering the costs involved in implementing each allocation method. When Ashley asked Jerry about the costs inherent in each allocation method, Jerry said, "I don't know! Assume that the direct method is the least costly, the reciprocal method is the most costly, and the other two fall somewhere in between." He also expects Ashley to make some judgments on the relative profitability of the patient services departments under the recommended allocation system.

Ashley began her analysis by reviewing the allocation methods presented in her old healthcare finance textbook. She had no problem remembering basic cost allocation concepts, but she did hit two snags. The first problem was that the textbook did not describe the double apportionment method. However, after a little research, Ashley discovered that the double apportionment method is a slightly more complicated version of the step-down method. In the first apportionment, support provided by each service department to the other service departments as well as to the patient services departments is recognized. Because some costs still remain in the support departments after the first apportionment, a second apportionment, which applies the step-down method, moves all remaining support department costs to the patient services departments. Thus, in the double apportionment method, service department support to all other service departments is recognized, while in the pure step-down method, service department support is recognized only to "downstream" service departments.

Here's how Ashley assumed that the double apportionment method would be applied to the Group. (There are alternative ways in which this allocation method can be applied.) First, direct Administration costs would be allocated to the other five departments (two support and three patient services). Second, direct Facilities costs would be allocated to all other departments (including Administration and Finance).

Third, direct Finance costs would be allocated to all other departments (including Administration and Facilities). After these three allocations are completed, the first apportionment is finished. Some costs remain in the support departments—the intrasupport department allocations from the first apportionment—so a second apportionment is necessary. The second apportionment is conducted using the step-down method as it is normally applied, except that the application of the first apportionment means that the starting cost pool values are much lower.

The second problem Ashley faced was that she did not know how to perform the reciprocal allocation. One method is to use simultaneous equations—but higher mathematics has never been Ashley's strong suit—and another method uses an iterative approach. Fortunately, Ashley had recently read an article in *Accounting Monthly* discussing an Excel model that uses the iterative approach to perform reciprocal allocation. To help with the analysis, Ashley modified the magazine's model by using the Group's numbers to calculate the allocation not only for the reciprocal method but also for the other three methods.

Assume that you are in Ashley's shoes. Complete her assignment and prepare a report to present to the Group's executive committee. In addition to merely completing the task as it stands, you decide to assess the sensitivity of the results to (1) the relative sizes of the direct costs at each support department and (2) the amount of support provided by the support departments to each other. Exhibit 4.3 contains the values that you intend to use in your sensitivity analysis.

EXHIBIT 4.1
Eagan Family Practice:
Departmental Revenue
and Cost Projections

Revenues	
Adult Medicine	$12,000,000
Obstetrics	6,000,000
Pediatrics	2,000,000
Total revenues	$20,000,000
Direct Costs	
Patient Services	
Adult Medicine	$ 6,000,000
Obstetrics	3,600,000
Pediatrics	1,200,000
Subtotal	$10,800,000
Support	
Administration	1,000,000
Facilities	4,400,000
Finance	1,800,000
Subtotal	$ 7,200,000
Total expenses	$18,000,000
Pretax profit	$ 2,000,000

	Percentage of Services Provided by		
Services Provided to	*Administration*	*Facilities*	*Finance*
Administration	—	5%	5%
Facilities	10%	—	5
Finance	10	10	—
Adult Medicine	35	55	50
Obstetrics	20	10	25
Pediatrics	25	20	15
Total	100%	100%	100%
Percentage to support departments	20%	15%	10%
Percentage to patient service departments	80%	85%	90%

EXHIBIT 4.2
Eagan Family Practice:
Allocation Percentages

Notes: 1. The allocation percentages are based on a two-year analysis of the actual services provided by the support departments to other departments.

2. To use the percentages to perform an allocation, they may have to be adjusted to ensure that the entire amount of the cost pool is allocated. To illustrate, in the direct method, all of Administration's costs ($500,000) have to be allocated directly in a single allocation to the three patient service departments. If the raw percentages were used, only 35% + 20% + 25% = 80% of the cost pool would be allocated, so the allocation percentages have to be adjusted so that 80 percent represents the entire allocation (100 percent). Thus, instead of a 35 percent allocation to Adult Medicine, its adjusted allocation is 35%/80% = 43.75%. In a similar manner, the adjusted allocation to Obstetrics is 20%/80% = 25%, while the adjusted allocation to Pediatrics is 25%/80% = 31.25%. When done correctly, the adjusted percentages must sum to 100%: 43.75% + 25% + 31.25% = 100%.

EXHIBIT 4.3
Eagan Family Practice:
Sensitivity Analysis
Values

Sensitivity to Changes in Relative Overhead Costs:

New Direct Expenses for Calculation 1

Administration	$4,400,000
Facilities	1,000,000
Finance	1,800,000
Total overhead expenses	$7,200,000

New Direct Expenses for Calculation 2

Administration	$1,000,000
Facilities	1,800,000
Finance	4,400,000
Total overhead expenses	$7,200,000

Sensitivity to Allocation Percentages:

	Percentage of Services Provided by		
Services Provided to	*Administration*	*Facilities*	*Finance*
Administration	—	25%	20%
Facilities	30%	—	20
Finance	30	25	—
Adult Medicine	18	32	33
Obstetrics	10	6	17
Pediatrics	12	12	10
Total	100%	100%	100%
Percentage to support departments	60%	50%	40%
Percentage to patient service departments	40%	50%	60%

NEW ENGLAND HEALTHCARE

PREMIUM DEVELOPMENT

5

NEW ENGLAND HEALTHCARE, a regional not-for-profit managed care company headquartered in Hartford, Connecticut, currently has more than 1 million enrollees in 25 different plans in Connecticut, Maine, Massachusetts, New Hampshire, Rhode Island, and Vermont. It has recently been contacted by a consortium of employers, including such major companies as IBM, GE, and Prudential, regarding its interest in bidding on a managed care (HMO) contract to be offered to the consortium's 75,000 employees and family members located in and around Nashua, New Hampshire.

New England's approach to premium development starts with the recognition that the premium received from employers must cover two different categories of expenses: (1) the cost of providing required healthcare services (medical costs) and (2) the costs of administering the plan and establishing reserves (other costs). Reserves, which typically are required by state insurance regulators, are necessary to ensure that funds are available to pay providers when medical costs exceed the amount collected in premium payments. New England, as a not-for-profit corporation, does not explicitly include a profit element in its premium. However, the reserve requirement is set sufficiently high that income from reserve investments is available to fund product expansion and growth; in effect, a portion of the reserve requirement constitutes profit.

New England uses a multistep approach in setting its premiums. First, a base per member per month (PMPM) cost is estimated for each of the plan's covered benefits. When the premiums are initially established for a new subscriber group, the base PMPM costs are usually developed on the basis of historical utilization and cost data. If data are available on the specific subscriber group, as with the consortium contract, these data are used. Otherwise, the base PMPM costs are based on utilization and cost data from one or more proxy groups, which are chosen to match as closely as possible the demographic, utilization, and cost patterns that will be experienced under the new contract. Also, any utilization or cost savings that will result from New England's aggressive utilization management program is factored into the premium.

The base PMPM costs then are adjusted to reflect the dollar amount of copayments to providers as well as the estimated impact of copayment and benefit options on utilization and hence medical costs. Copayments, which are an additional source of revenue to the provider panel, reduce New England's medical costs and thus lower the consortium's premium. Furthermore, the higher the copayment, the lower the utilization of that service, especially if it is noncritical. Finally, the more restrictive the benefits package, the lower the costs associated with medical services. The end result, after these adjustments are made, is an adjusted PMPM cost for each service, which are then summed to obtain the total medical PMPM amount.

To estimate the total nonmedical PMPM amount, New England typically adds 15 percent to the total medical PMPM amount for administrative costs and 5 percent for reserves. The sum of the total medical and total nonmedical amounts, which is called the "total PMPM amount," is the per member amount that New England must collect from the consortium each month to meet the total costs of serving the healthcare needs of its employees—the subscribers to the plan.

Once the total PMPM amount is calculated, it must be converted into actual premium rates for individuals and families. Using data provided by the consortium, New England estimates that 45 percent of subscribers will elect individual coverage, while the remaining 55 percent will choose family coverage. New England plans to offer the consortium a two-rate structure, under which employees may elect either single or family coverage. Data from the consortium indicate that family coverage, on average, includes 3.5 individuals, so, all else the same, the premiums for families should be 3.5 times as much as for individuals. However, children typically consume less healthcare services, on a dollar basis, than do adults, so final premiums must reflect such differentials.

Here are the factor rates for obtaining individual and family premium rates:

Single factor: 1.216   Family factor: 3.356

In setting the specific premium rates, New England must ensure that the total premiums collected, which would be paid by both the employer and employees, equal the estimated total calculated using the PMPM rate. The 75,000 population who would be served by the contract consists (roughly) of 12,000 individual members and 18,000 families. Thus, 75,000 × Total PMPM amount must equal (12,000 × Single premium) + (18,000 × Family premium).

Exhibit 5.1 is a partially completed copy of the worksheet that New England uses to establish the total PMPM amount and premium rates on any contract. The worksheet provides a relatively easy guide for implementing the procedures described above. Exhibit 5.2 contains the relevant cost and utilization adjustment factors for a variety of service and copayment options. Once the decision has been made on the appropriate service and copay structure, these adjustment factors feed into the calculations in Exhibit 5.1 for each service's medical PMPM amount.

The consortium has furnished New England with a significant amount of data concerning its employees' current utilization of healthcare services. The inpatient cost and utilization data for consortium employees are as follows:

Average daily fee-for-service charge $1,400
Utilization ($100 copay)   500 days per year per 1,000 members

Note, however, that a recent survey of New Hampshire hospitals indicates that most managed care contracts call for per diem payments in the range of $1,000 to $1,200. Additionally, New England's experience with similar employee groups indicates that moderate utilization management would result in 400–450 inpatient days per 1,000 plan members.

Exhibit 5.3 shows current cost and utilization data for other facility services, including skilled nursing care, inpatient mental health care, hospital surgical services, and emergency department care. The utilization and cost data on primary care services for consortium employees are as follows:

Current number of visits ($5 copay)	3.4 per year per member

New England routinely pays primary care physicians a capitated amount based on annual costs of $200,000. It assumes that one primary care physician can handle 4,000 patient visits per year. Utilization and cost data for specialist office visits are as follows:

Current number of visits ($0 copay)	1.5 per year per member
Current cost per visit	$92.65

Note that the total PMPM amount shown in Exhibit 5.1 may be modified to reflect anticipated medical cost inflation. This adjustment is especially critical if the total PMPM premium is based on relatively old cost data. For the most part, the cost data provided in the case can be assumed to be two years old (the data are for last year, and the contract would not be in place for yet another year).

Also, note that the premium calculation in Exhibit 5.1 does not include certain medical services, such as routine vision and dental care, chiropractic services, durable medical equipment, out-of-network services, and pharmacy benefits. The consortium specifically requested that the initial premium bid exclude such "rider" services. However, if New England is chosen to submit a final premium bid, the consortium will likely request pricing on one or more riders.

Finally, with no guidance from the consortium regarding the level of services desired or the copay structure, New England intends to offer three choices to the consortium: low cost, moderate cost, and high cost. Of course, these plans differ in that the low-cost (to the consortium) plan requires higher copays by employees and has more limitations on covered services; the high-cost plan has lower copays and fewer limitations; and the moderate-cost plan falls between the two extremes.

Assume that you have recently joined New England Healthcare as a marketing analyst. Your first task is to develop the bid presentation to be made to the consortium. (**Note: The data in this case are for illustrative purposes only and do not reflect current healthcare costs.**)

I. Medical Expenses

	Base PMPM Cost	Copay Adjustment Factors		Adjusted PMPM
		Cost	*Utilization*	
Facility Services				
Inpatient:				
Acute	$			$
Skilled nursing				
Mental health				
Substance abuse	0.41	1.0000	1.0000	0.41
Surgical procedures				
Emergency department				
Outpatient procedures	3.43	1.0000	1.0000	3.43
Total facilities				
Physician Services				
Primary care services				
Specialist services:				
Office visits				
Surgical services	9.00	0.9544	1.0000	8.59
All other services	23.67	0.8659	0.9100	18.65
Total physicians				
Total medical PMPM amount				

II. Nonmedical Expenses

Administrative

Reserves

Total nonmedical PMPM amount

III. Total Expenses

Total PMPM amount

IV. Premium Rates

	Single	*Family*
Rate factor		
Premium rate		

EXHIBIT 5.1
New England Healthcare:
Premium Development
Worksheet

EXHIBIT 5.2
New England Healthcare:
Cost and Utilization
Adjustment Factors

	Patient Copay Amount	Copay Cost Adj. Factor	Copay Utilization Adj. Factor
Facility Services			
Inpatient acute	$ 0	1.0000	1.0000
	100	0.9851	0.9750
	150	0.9777	0.9600
	250	0.9642	0.9200
Skilled nursing	$ 0	1.0000	1.0000
Mental health:			
30-day limit	$ 0	1.0000	0.9524
	100	0.9805	0.9286
	150	0.9707	0.9143
	250	0.9532	0.8762
60-day limit	$ 0	1.0000	1.2000
	100	0.9845	1.1700
	150	0.9768	1.1520
	250	0.9628	1.1040
90-day limit	$ 0	1.0000	1.2500
	100	0.9851	1.2188
	150	0.9777	1.2000
	250	0.9643	1.1500
Surgical procedures	$ 0	1.0000	1.0000
	100	0.9231	1.0000
	150	0.8846	1.0000
	250	0.8077	1.0000
Emergency department	$ 0	1.0857	1.0250
	15	1.0000	1.0000
	25	0.9429	0.9850
	50	0.8000	0.9550

	Patient Copay Amount	Copay Cost Adj. Factor	Copay Utilization Adj. Factor
Primary Care Services	$ 0	1.0352	1.0150
	5	1.0000	1.0000
	10	0.9472	0.9800
	15	0.8593	0.9500
	20	0.7713	0.9200
	25	0.6834	0.8900
Specialist Services			
Zero PCP copay	$ 0	1.0000	1.0000
	5	0.8897	0.9730
	10	0.7795	0.9590
	15	0.6692	0.9450
$10 PCP copay	$ 0	1.0000	0.9920
	5	0.8897	0.9600
	10	0.7795	0.9460
	15	0.6692	0.9320
$20 PCP copay	$ 0	1.0000	0.9680
	5	0.8897	0.9360
	10	0.7795	0.9220
	15	0.6692	0.9080

**EXHIBIT 5.2
(continued)
New England Healthcare:
Cost and Utilization
Adjustment Factors**

PCP: primary care physician

Note: New England uses various incentive systems to control utilization of specialty services. One system requires PCPs to assess a copay for each specialist office visit.

EXHIBIT 5.3
Consortium Employee
Utilization and Cost Data:
Other Facility Services

Skilled nursing facility care	25.2 days per year per 1,000 members
Current average daily cost	$650
Inpatient mental health care ($0 copay)	64.4 days per year per 1,000 members
Current average daily cost	$740
Hospital-based surgery ($0 copay)	41.7 cases per year per 1,000 members
Current costs	$1,800 per case
Emergency department care ($15 copay)	132 visits per year per 1,000 members
Current costs	$250 per visit (see note)

Note: The emergency department cost is the total charge for facility services, some of which would be covered by the $15 copay.

TULSA MEMORIAL HOSPITAL

6

BREAK-EVEN ANALYSIS

TULSA MEMORIAL HOSPITAL (TMH), an acute care hospital with 300 beds and 160 staff physicians, is one of 75 hospitals owned and operated by Health Services of America, a for-profit, publicly owned company. Although there are nine other acute care hospitals serving the same general population, TMH historically has been highly profitable because of its well-appointed facilities, its fine medical staff, its reputation for quality care, and the amount of individual attention it gives to its patients. In addition to inpatient services, TMH operates an emergency department within the hospital complex and a stand-alone urgent care center located across the street from the area's major shopping mall, about two miles from the hospital.

According to a *Wall Street Journal* article, urgent care centers are increasingly visited by patients who need immediate treatment for an illness, such as the flu or a sore throat, or an injury, such as a nail-gun wound. Urgent care centers are distinguished from similar types of ambulatory healthcare providers, such as emergency departments and retail clinics, by the scope of illnesses treated and the presence of on-site facilities. These centers help mitigate the problems of primary care physician shortages and already crowded (and typically very expensive) emergency departments.

Urgent care centers, notes the *Wall Street Journal* article, are staffed by physicians, offer short wait times, and charge between $60 and $200 per procedure. Furthermore, no appointments are necessary and evening and weekend hours are frequently available. Finally, many centers offer discounts to the uninsured, and for those with coverage, copayments are

47

typically much less than for emergency department visits. There are currently about 9,000 of these centers around the country, including about 1,500 that are hospital affiliated.

The Urgent Care Association of America has established criteria for designation as a Certified Urgent Care Center. Currently, about half of the centers in the United States have this certification. According to MedLibrary.org, "these criteria define scope of service, hours of operation, and staffing requirements. A qualifying facility must accept walk-in patients of all ages during all hours of operation. It should treat a 'broad-spectrum' of illnesses and injuries, and have the ability to perform minor procedures. An urgent care center must also have on-site diagnostic services, including phlebotomy and x-ray." (For more information on urgent care centers, see www.ucaoa.org.) In addition to certification, urgent care centers can obtain accreditation through The Joint Commission as part of its ambulatory healthcare accreditation program. (For more information, see www.jointcommission.org.)

Brandon Harley, TMH's chief executive officer, is concerned about the urgent care center's overall financial soundness. About ten years ago, several area hospitals jumped onto the urgent care center bandwagon, and within a short time, there were 15 such centers scattered around the city. Now, only 11 are left, and none of them appears to be a big moneymaker. Brandon wonders if TMH should continue to operate its center or close it down. The center is currently handling a patient load of 45 visits per day, but it has the physical capacity to handle many more—up to 85 visits a day. Brandon's decision is complicated by the fact that Amanda Daniels, TMH's marketing director, has been pushing to embark on a new marketing program for the clinic. She believes that an expanded marketing effort aimed at local businesses would bring in the number of new patients needed to make the clinic a financial winner.

Brandon has asked Nicole Williams, TMH's chief financial officer, to look into the whole matter of the urgent care center. In their meeting, Brandon stated that he visualizes three potential outcomes for the center: (1) it could be closed; (2) it could continue to operate as is—that is, without expanding its marketing program; or (3) it could continue to operate, accompanied by the expanded marketing effort. As a starting point for the analysis, Nicole collected the most recent historical financial and operating data for the center, which are summarized in Exhibit 6.1. In assessing the historical data, she noted that one competing center had recently (December 2013) closed its doors. Furthermore, a review of several years of financial data revealed that TMH's urgent care center does not have a pronounced seasonal utilization pattern.

Next, Nicole met several times with the center's administrative director. The primary purpose of the meetings was to estimate the additional costs that would have to be borne if center volume rose above the current January/February average level of 45 visits per day. Any incremental usage would require additional expenditures for administrative and medical supplies, estimated to be $4.00 per patient visit for medical supplies, such as tongue blades and rubber gloves, and $1.00 per patient visit for administrative supplies, such as file folders and clinical record sheets.

Because of the relatively low volume level, the urgent care center has purposely been staffed at the bare minimum. In fact, some center employees have started to grumble about not being able to do their jobs well because of overwork. Thus, any increase in the number of patient visits would require immediate administrative and medical staffing increases. Furthermore, as the number of visits increase, the center would have to hire additional staff members. The incremental costs associated with increased volume are summarized in Exhibit 6.2.

The urgent care center's building is leased on a long-term basis. TMH could cancel the lease, but the lease contract calls for a cancelation penalty of three months' rent, or $37,500 at the current lease rate. In addition, Nicole was startled to read in the newspaper that Baptist Hospital, TMH's major competitor, had just bought the city's largest primary care practice, and Baptist's CEO was quoted as saying that more group practice acquisitions are planned as the hospital moved to embrace healthcare reform. Nicole wondered whether Baptist's actions would influence the decision regarding the urgent care center's fate.

Finally, Nicole met with Amanda to learn more about the proposed marketing program. The primary focus of the new marketing program would be on occupational health services (OHS). OHS involves providing medical care to local businesses, including physical examinations for managers and employees; treatment of illnesses that occur during working hours; and treatment of work-related injuries, especially those covered by workers' compensation. Although some of the clinic's current business is OHS related, Amanda believes that a strong marketing effort, coupled with specialized OHS record keeping, could bring additional patients to the clinic. The proposed marketing expansion requires a marketing assistant who will run the clinic's OHS program. Additionally, the new marketing program would incur advertising costs for newspaper, radio, and TV ads as well as for brochures and handouts. The incremental costs associated with the new marketing program are also summarized in Exhibit 6.2. (To learn more about OHS, start at the American College of Occupational and Environmental Medicine website, www.acoem.org.)

With a blank spreadsheet on her computer screen, Nicole began to construct a model that would provide the information needed to help the board make a rational, informed decision. At first, Nicole planned to conduct a standard capital budgeting analysis that focused on the profitability of the clinic as measured by net present value or internal rate of return. Then she realized that the expanded marketing program requires no capital investment. She also realized that no valid data are available on the incremental increase in visits that would be generated by either an increasing population base or the expanded marketing program. Finally, she remembered that Brandon requested that the analysis consider the inherent profitability of the clinic without the expanded marketing program.

With these points in mind, Nicole thought that a break-even analysis would be very useful in making the final decision. Specifically, she wanted to develop answers to the following questions posed by Brandon:

1. What is the projected profitability of the urgent care center for the entire year if volume continues at its current level?
2. How many additional visits per day would be required to break even without the new marketing program?
3. How many additional visits per day would be required to break even assuming that the new marketing program is undertaken?
4. How many additional daily visits would the new program have to bring in to make it worthwhile, regardless of the overall profitability of the clinic?

In addition, Nicole wondered if the clinic could "inflate" its way to profitability; that is, if volume remained at its current level, could the clinic be expected to become profitable in, say, five years, solely because of inflationary increases in revenues? Finally, Nicole was concerned whether or not the analysis was giving the clinic full credit for its financial contributions to the hospital. She did not want to change the spreadsheet at this late date, but she did want to make sure that any additional financial value was at least considered qualitatively. Overall, Nicole must consider all relevant factors—both quantitative and qualitative—and come up with a recommendation regarding the future of the urgent care center.

EXHIBIT 6.1
TMH Urgent Care Center:
Historical Financial Data

	CY 2013	Jan 2014	Feb 2014	Monthly Averages 2013	Monthly Averages Jan/Feb 2014	Total
Number of visits	14,522	1,365	1,335	1,210	1,350	1,230
Net revenue	$548,747	$55,028	$54,748	$45,729	$54,888	$47,037
Salaries and wages	$154,250	$13,540	$13,544	$12,854	$13,542	$12,952
Physician fees	192,000	18,000	18,000	16,000	18,000	16,286
Malpractice insurance	31,440	3,215	3,215	2,620	3,215	2,705
Travel and education	5,365	538	665	447	602	469
General insurance	8,112	843	843	676	843	700
Subscriptions	189	0	0	16	0	14
Electricity	11,820	1,124	1,029	985	1,077	998
Water	1,260	135	142	105	139	110
Equipment rental	1,260	105	105	105	105	105
Building lease	155,745	12,500	12,500	12,979	12,500	12,910
Other operating expenses	103,779	8,152	7,923	8,648	8,038	8,561
Total operating expenses	$665,220	$58,152	$57,966	$55,435	$58,059	$55,810
Net profit (loss)	($116,473)	($ 3,124)	($ 3,218)	($ 9,706)	($ 3,173)	($ 8,773)
Gross margin (%)	−21.2%	−5.7%	−5.9%	−21.2%	−5.8%	−18.7%

CY: current year

	Number of Additional Visits per Day					
	0	1–10	11–20	21–30	31–40	

EXHIBIT 6.2
TMH Urgent Care Center:
Monthly Incremental
Cost Data

Variable Costs

Medical supplies — $4.00 per visit

Administrative supplies — 1.00 per visit

Total variable costs per visit — $5.00 per visit

Semifixed Costs

	0	1–10	11–20	21–30	31–40
Salaries and wages		$ 5,000	$ 6,000	$ 7,000	$ 8,000
Physician fees		12,000	12,000	12,000	16,000
Total monthly semifixed costs	$ 0	$17,000	$18,000	$19,000	$24,000

Fixed Costs

	0	1–10	11–20	21–30	31–40
Marketing assistant's salary	$ 3,000	$ 3,000	$ 3,000	$ 3,000	$ 3,000
Advertising expenses	4,000	4,000	4,000	4,000	4,000
Total monthly fixed costs	$ 7,000	$ 7,000	$ 7,000	$ 7,000	$ 7,000

CASCADES MENTAL HEALTH CLINIC

VARIANCE ANALYSIS

7

CASCADES MENTAL HEALTH Clinic is a not-for-profit, multidisciplinary mental health provider that offers both inpatient and outpatient services on a full-risk (capitated) basis to members of managed care plans. Its clinical staff consists primarily of psychiatrists, psychologists, psychiatric nurses, social workers, and chemical dependency counselors. Currently, Cascades has major contracts with two large managed care organizations in its service area: Pacific Care and Seattle Healthplans. Each of these organizations has both commercial and Medicare health maintenance organization (HMO) contracts with Cascades. Thus, in total, there are four separate product lines.

Cascades is partially funded by state and local government. The agreement with the funding agencies is that funds received are to be used to cover overhead and capital expenses. Furthermore, expenses for drugs and other medical and administrative supplies are billed separately to the HMOs at cost. Thus, overhead and supplies expenses are not part of this budget, which means that the analysis focuses on clinical labor expenses. If the assumption is made that other payment mechanisms cover overhead, capital expenses, and supplies at cost, then Cascades' profitability is solely a function of its ability to create revenues that exceed labor costs. Thus, its operating budget focuses on enrollment, per member premiums, utilization, and labor costs.

Exhibit 7.1 lists the assumptions used to prepare Cascades' 2013 operating budget. Note that the four product lines are expected to provide a total of 4,551,000 member-months of revenue during 2013. Also, note that each product line has a different per member per month

55

(PMPM) payment (premium) amount. Exhibit 7.1 also shows expected admission (for inpatients), referral rate (for outpatients), and labor cost and utilization data for each product line. Because of the unique employment arrangements between Cascades and its clinical staff, in which the staff are paid on the basis of the number of patient service units provided, clinical labor costs are virtually all variable, and hence labor costs are not identified as fixed or variable.

Exhibit 7.2 contains the forecasted 2013 budget. In essence, data from Exhibit 7.1 are used to forecast revenues and costs, both in the aggregate and by product line. Overall, Cascades expected to earn a total profit of $419,379 on the four product lines in 2013.

During the first quarter of 2013, Cascades' managers noted a higher utilization rate than budgeted. To add to their concern, the monthly enrollment figures supplied by the contracting managed care plans were less than those budgeted. Together, these trends indicated lower revenues and higher per enrollee costs, and hence lower profits, than forecasted in Exhibit 7.2. These concerns were borne out when the first-quarter profits came in under budget. To help stem the adverse trend, Cascades' managers instituted a utilization management system in which all inpatient stays were required to be approved by the clinic's medical director—a senior staff psychiatrist. In addition, Cascades was able to make midyear changes to its commercial premiums that increased the average premiums for the year.

Unfortunately, the action taken was "too little, too late" to save the year. Exhibit 7.3 provides operating results for 2013, while Exhibit 7.4 shows the realized aggregate and product line profit and loss (P&L) statements. A quick review of Exhibit 7.4 reveals that the signals conveyed by the first-quarter data were indeed correct; although 2013 ended with a profit, the profit was much less than the amount forecasted.

When the results were submitted to Cascades' CEO, Jennifer Jacobs, she grimaced and said, "I knew it was coming, but I did not expect the profit number to be so low." It was immediately apparent to Jennifer that Cascades could not afford similar results in 2014. She knew that something had to be done, but the best course of action was not clear.

To help plan for next year, Jennifer asked Cascades' finance and accounting department head, Rob Maldonado, to perform a variance analysis on the data to help identify the problems that led to the poor financial results for 2013. Unfortunately, Rob's area of expertise is dealing with lenders and other capital suppliers, so he passed the assignment on to you, a newly hired financial analyst.

To start the analysis, you created a diagram (Exhibit 7.5) to help understand variance analysis. (Note that this diagram is generic in nature and has not been "customized" for this case.) Furthermore, you recognize that because the volume variance consists of differences in both enrollment and utilization, it is necessary to create two flexible budgets: one flexed (adjusted) for actual enrollment only and the other flexed for both actual enrollment and actual utilization. Additionally, to help with the calculations, you jotted down an equation list for calculating variances. (Note that not all of the equations listed are necessarily applicable to this analysis.) This list is contained in Exhibit 7.6.

Of course, both Jennifer and Rob are more concerned with what the numbers mean than what the numbers are. Therefore, your variance analysis should include a great deal of interpretation along with the numbers. Finally, you would like to use this assignment to help advance your career within the organization, so you plan to go one step further by offering recommendations for management action along with the numbers and interpretation.

**EXHIBIT 7.1
Cascades Mental Health
Clinic: 2013 Operating
Budget Assumptions**

Expected Enrollment (member-months)

PC Commercial	3,365,000
PC Medicare	469,000
SH Commercial	502,000
SH Medicare	215,000
Total	4,551,000

Expected Premium Data (per member per month)

PC Commercial	$0.70
PC Medicare	0.85
SH Commercial	0.75
SH Medicare	0.80

Expected Labor Data per Admission or Session

	Inpatient		Outpatient	
	No. of Hours	Hourly Rate	No. of Hours	Hourly Rate
PC Commercial	53.74	$35	1.04	$100
PC Medicare	68.43	35	1.30	100
SH Commercial	47.77	35	1.15	100
SH Medicare	56.86	35	1.14	100

Expected Utilization and Total Labor Cost Data

Plan Type	Avg No. of Members (in 000s)	Inpatient				Outpatient			Total
		Admission Rate	Cost per Admission	Total Costs	Referral Rate	Cost per Session	Total Costs		
PC:									
Commercial	280.417	3.81	$1,881	$2,009,639	2.00	$104	$58,327		$2,067,966
Medicare	39.083	3.96	2,395	370,671	2.00	130	10,162		380,833
Total	319.500			$2,380,310			$68,489		$2,448,799
SH:									
Commercial	41.833	3.89	$1,672	$ 272,085	2.00	$115	$ 9,622		$ 281,707
Medicare	17.917	4.17	1,990	148,681	2.00	114	4,085		152,766
Total	59.750			$ 420,766			$13,707		$ 434,473
Grand total	379.250			$2,801,076			$82,196		$2,883,272

PC: Pacific Care; SH: Seattle Healthplans

EXHIBIT 7.1
(continued)
Cascades Mental Health
Clinic: 2013 Operating
Budget Assumptions

**EXHIBIT 7.2
Cascades Mental
Health Clinic:
2013 Operating Budget**

Expected Product Line and Aggregate Profits

	PC		SH		
	Commercial	Medicare	Commercial	Medicare	Total
Revenue	$2,335,500	$ 398,650	$ 376,500	$172,000	$3,302,650
Costs	2,067,964	380,836	281,709	152,763	2,883,271
Profit	$ 287,536	$ 17,814	$ 94,791	$ 19,237	$ 419,379
Margin	12.3%	4.5%	25.2%	11.2%	12.7%

**EXHIBIT 7.3
Cascades Mental
Health Clinic:
2013 Operating Results**

Actual Enrollment (member-months)

PC Commercial	3,073,133
PC Medicare	485,000
SH Commercial	547,105
SH Medicare	257,000
Total	4,362,238

Actual Premium Data (per member per month)

PC Commercial	$0.75
PC Medicare	0.85
SH Commercial	0.80
SH Medicare	0.80

Actual Labor Data per Admission or Session

	Inpatient		Outpatient	
	No. of Hours	Hourly Rate	No. of Hours	Hourly Rate
PC Commercial	47.32	$38	0.95	$109.50
PC Medicare	58.66	38	1.15	109.50
SH Commercial	52.06	33	0.98	95
SH Medicare	84.85	33	2.00	95

Actual Utilization and Cost Data

Plan Type	Avg No. of Members (in 000s)	Inpatient			Referral Rate	Outpatient		Total
		Admission Rate	Cost per Admission	Total Costs		Cost per Session	Total Costs	
PC:								
Commercial	256.094	4.33	$1,798	$1,993,782	3.65	$104	$ 97,213	$2,090,996
Medicare	40.417	4.68	2,229	421,615	1.86	126	9,472	431,087
Total	296.511			$2,415,397			$106,685	$2,522,083
SH:								
Commercial	45.592	5.79	$1,718	$ 453,514	3.35	$ 93	$ 14,204	$ 467,719
Medicare	21.417	4.56	2,800	273,448	1.75	190	7,121	280,569
Total	67.009			$ 726,962			$ 21,325	$ 748,288
Grand total	363.520			$3,142,360			$128,011	$3,270,371

Note: These data were generated on a spreadsheet, and hence some rounding differences occur.

EXHIBIT 7.3
(continued)
Cascades Mental
Health Clinic:
2013 Operating Results

**EXHIBIT 7.4
Cascades Mental
Health Clinic:
2013 Actual P&L
Statements**

Product Line and Aggregate Profit Results

	PC		SH		
	Commercial	*Medicare*	*Commercial*	*Medicare*	*Total*
Revenue	$2,304,850	$ 412,250	$ 437,684	$205,600	$3,360,384
Costs	2,090,996	431,087	467,719	280,569	3,270,371
Profit	$ 213,584	($ 18,837)	($ 30,035)	($ 74,969)	$ 90,013
Margin	9.3%	(4.6%)	(6.9%)	(36.5%)	2.7%

Note: These data were generated on a spreadsheet, and hence some rounding differences occur.

**EXHIBIT 7.5
Variance Analysis
Summary**

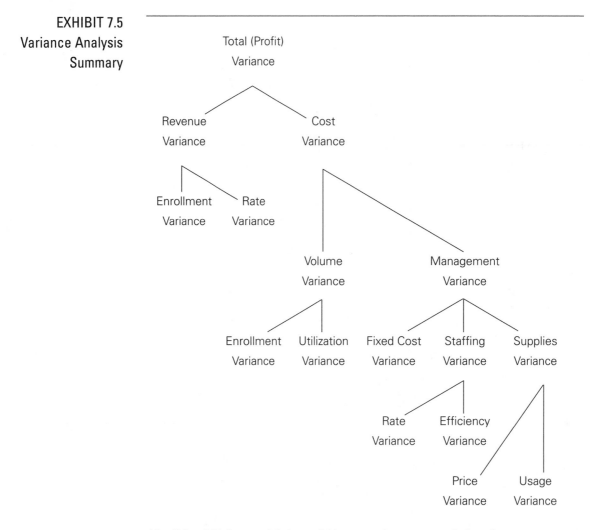

Hint: This exhibit format might be useful for presenting your numerical results.

EXHIBIT 7.6
Generic Equation List

Total variance	= Actual profit − Static profit
Revenue variance	= Actual revenue − Static revenue
Enrollment variance	= Flexible (enrollment) revenue − Static revenue
Rate variance	= Actual revenue − Flexible (enrollment) revenue
Cost variance	= Static costs − Actual costs
Volume variance	= Static costs − Flexible (enrollment/utilization) costs
Enrollment variance	= Static costs − Flexible (enrollment) costs
Utilization variance	= Flexible (enrollment) costs − Flexible (enrollment/ utilization) costs
Management variance	= Flexible (enrollment/utilization) costs − Actual costs
Fixed cost variance	= Actual fixed costs − Flexible fixed costs
Staffing variance	= Actual staffing costs − Flexible (enrollment/utilization) staffing costs
Rate variance	= (Static hourly labor rate − Actual hourly labor rate) x Actual number of hours per episode x Actual utilization rate x Actual enrollment
Efficiency variance	= (Expected number of hours per episode − Actual number of hours per episode) x Expected hourly labor rate x Actual utilization rate x Actual enrollment
Supplies variance	= Flexible (enrollment/utilization) supplies costs − Actual supplies costs
Price variance	= (Static price − Actual price) x Actual units
Usage variance	= (Flexible units − Actual units) x Static price

Note: Not all of the above equations are necessarily useful to all product lines.

MOUNTAIN VILLAGE CLINIC

CASH BUDGETING

8

MOUNTAIN VILLAGE CLINIC is a small walk-in clinic adjacent to the primary ski area of Mountain Village, a winter resort located a short distance from Aspen, Colorado. It should be no surprise that the clinic specializes in the treatment of injuries sustained while skiing. It is owned and operated by two physicians: James Peterson, an orthopedist, and Amanda Cook, an internist. Patient volume at the clinic is highly seasonal because the vast majority of the business occurs during the ski season, which generally runs from December through March. In fact, at one time Drs. Peterson and Cook thought about closing the clinic during the slow months, but (1) the clinic would be very difficult to operate efficiently for only a portion of the year and (2) the area has started to attract a sizable amount of summer visitors, which has made summer operations more financially attractive.

The clinic has an outside accountant who takes care of payroll matters, but Dr. Cook does all the other financial work for the clinic. However, to help in that task, the clinic recently hired a part-time MHA student, Doug Washington. On a Wednesday afternoon in October 2013, Dr. Cook called Doug into her office to tell him about an upcoming meeting with the head of commercial lending at First Bank of Aspen, the clinic's primary lender. The purpose of the meeting is to discuss cash management services and the clinic's line-of-credit requirements. A line of credit is a short-term loan agreement by which a bank agrees to lend a business some specified maximum amount. The business can borrow (draw down) against the credit line at any time it is in force, which typically is no longer than one year.

When a line expires, it must be renegotiated if it is still needed. The amount borrowed on the line, or some lesser amount, can be repaid at any time, but any amount outstanding must be repaid at expiration. Interest is charged daily on the amount drawn down, and a commitment fee often is required up front to secure the line. In general, lines of credit are used by businesses to meet temporary (usually seasonal) cash needs, as opposed to being used for permanent long-term financing. Currently, the interest rate on First Bank line-of-credit draw-downs is 4 percent compounded monthly (4%/12 = 0.333% per month), and First Bank pays 2 percent compounded monthly (2%/12 = 0.167% per month) on temporary investments of excess cash. Interest earned (paid) occurs in the month following the end-of-month cash surplus (loan requirement).

To prepare for the upcoming meeting with the bank, Dr. Cook asked Doug to develop a cash budget and determine the line-of-credit amount the clinic should request. No one had taken the time to prepare a cash budget recently, although a spreadsheet model that had been constructed a few years ago was available for use. From information previously developed, Doug knew that no seasonal financing would be needed from First Bank before January, so he decided to restrict his budget to the period of January through June 2014.

As a first step, he looked through the clinic's financial records to get the data needed to develop the billings forecast, which is contained in Exhibit 8.1. To start, Doug assumed that actual billings as a percentage of forecast would be 100 percent. On the basis of the clinic's previous collections experience, Doug was able to convert billings for medical services into actual cash collections. On average, about 20 percent of the clinic's patients pay immediately for services rendered. Third-party payers pay the remaining claims, with 20 percent of the payments made within 30 days and the remaining 60 percent (of total billings) paid within 60 days.

Variable medical costs at the clinic are assumed to consist entirely of medical and administrative supplies. These supplies, which are estimated to cost 15 percent of billings, are purchased two months before expected usage. On average, the clinic pays about half of its suppliers in the month of purchase (two months before use) and the other half in the following month (one month before use).

Clinical labor costs (for physicians and other clinical employees) are the primary expense of the clinic. During the high season (December through March), these costs run $150,000 a month, but some of the clinical staff work only seasonally, so clinical labor costs drop to $120,000 a month in the remaining months.

The clinic pays fixed general and administrative expenses, including clerical labor, of approximately $30,000 a month, while lease obligations amount to $12,000 per month. These expenditures are expected to continue at the same level throughout the forecast period. The clinic's monthly miscellaneous expenses are estimated to be $10,000.

The clinic has a semi-annual, five-year, 10 percent, $500,000 term loan outstanding with First Bank for which payments of $64,752 are due on March 15 and September 15. Also, the clinic is planning to replace an old x-ray machine (which has no salvage value) in February with a new one that costs $125,000. The clinic is a partnership, so, for tax purposes, any profits (or losses) are prorated to the two physician partners, who must pay individual taxes on this income. Thus, no tax payments are built into the clinic's cash budget.

The clinic has to maintain a minimum cash balance of $50,000 at First Bank because of compensating balance requirements on its term loan. This amount, but no more, is expected to be on hand on January 1, 2014.

For the daily cash budget, Doug made some additional assumptions about volume and collections:

- The clinic operates seven days a week.
- Patient volume is more or less constant throughout the month, so the daily billings forecast will be 1/(Number of days in the month) multiplied by the billings forecast for that month.
- Daily billings follow the 20 percent–20 percent–60 percent collection breakdown based on monthly billings.
- Patient payments are assumed to occur on the day of billing, "early" payers are assumed to pay 30 days after billing, and "late" payers are assumed to pay 60 days after billing.
- The lease payment is made on the 1st of the month.
- Fifty percent of both clinical labor costs and general and administrative expenses are paid on the 1st of the month, and 50 percent are paid on the 15th of the month.

- Supplies are delivered on the 1st of the month and paid for on the 5th of the month.
- Miscellaneous expenses are incurred and paid evenly throughout each month.
- Term loan payments are made on the 15th of the month in which they are due.
- The compensating balance of $50,000 must be in the bank on each day.

Place yourself in Doug's position. Be prepared to discuss your analysis with Dr. Cook when you meet with her next week.

EXHIBIT 8.1
Mountain Village Clinic:
Billings Forecast

Year	Month	Amount
2013	November	$150,000
	December	250,000
2014	January	350,000
	February	450,000
	March	300,000
	April	150,000
	May	100,000
	June	175,000
	July	250,000
	August	200,000

CAMBRIDGE TRANSPLANT CENTER

MARGINAL COST PRICING ANALYSIS

9

CAMBRIDGE TRANSPLANT CENTER (the Center), which is part of University Healthcare System (the System), is a regional leader in the very intense and medically sophisticated area of organ transplantation. All transplants are performed at Cambridge General Hospital, the 400-bed flagship of the System.

The administrative director of the Center, Josh Zimmerman, has been on the job for ten years, during which time significant growth has occurred in both the number of transplant programs and the volume of procedures performed. When Josh joined the Center, he was put in charge of a kidney transplant program that averaged 60 transplants per year and a heart transplant program that performed 40 transplants annually. Today, the Center performs more than 500 transplants per year, including transplants from liver, lung, and pancreas programs.

The liver transplant program is the most successful of all the Center's organ programs in terms of volume and revenues. Last year, volume totaled 120 transplants, bringing in more than $50 million in total revenues. This year, Josh is optimistic that the liver program can do even better. However, he knows that increased volume is largely dependent on the number of organ donors and on his success in negotiating a new contract with Lifecare Transplant Network (LTNET), the largest transplant-benefits company in the nation.

Although most health insurers can identify those patients who are good candidates for transplant services, only the largest health insurers have the expertise to manage the transplant process. Transplants are relatively rare compared with other, more conventional medical procedures. However, the costs to insurers for transplant services are typically very large — usually in the six- to seven-figure range. To ensure the best and most cost-effective management of transplant services, most insurers outsource transplant management to companies, such as LTNET, that specialize in these services.

Contracting for transplant services is unique and complex because of the sophistication of the medical procedures involved. Transplant services consist of five phases: (1) patient evaluation, (2) patient care while awaiting surgery, (3) organ procurement, (4) surgery and the attendant inpatient stay, and (5) one year of follow-up visits. The costs involved in Phase 1 are relatively simple to estimate, but the remaining phases can be extremely variable in terms of resource utilization, and hence costs, because of differences in patient acuity and surgical outcomes.

Historically, reimbursement for transplant services has been handled in a number of different ways. Initially, many transplant providers bundled all five phases together and offered insurers a single, global rate. Although this method simplified the contracting process, the rate set was often chosen more on the basis of building market share than on covering costs. Indeed, many institutions could not even estimate with any confidence the true costs of providing transplant services.

Somewhat ironically, success in gaining market share usually increases the financial risk of the transplant program because higher volumes increase the likelihood of attracting higher-acuity patients. Furthermore, changes in the organ allocation system have promoted the acceptance of sicker patients into transplant programs. Although the total costs associated with all phases of a liver transplant average about $500,000, the amount can more than quadruple if the patient requires a re-transplant or if other complications occur. Because of this extreme variability in costs, outlier protection is a critical aspect of contract negotiations if the reimbursement methodology is a fixed prospective rate such as a global rate.

The LTNET contract requires the approval of Dr. Anjali Desai, the newly appointed surgical director of the liver transplant program. Fortunately, Dr. Desai shares Josh's enthusiasm to build the liver program into one of the largest in the country and, like Josh, is very motivated to secure the contract. In his second meeting with Dr. Desai, Josh discussed the specifics of the current contract negotiations. Phases 1, 2, and 5 will be reimbursed at a set discount from charges. Furthermore, to reduce the amount of financial risk borne by the Center, Phase 3 (organ procurement) will be reimbursed on a cost basis. This makes sense because the cost of Phase 3 is almost completely uncontrollable by the Center. Thus, the primary focus of the negotiations, and the make-or-break part of the contract, is the reimbursement amount for Phase 4. (For more information on organ procurement, see the United Network for Organ Sharing website at www.unos.org.)

Phase 4 costs are divided into two categories: hospital costs and physician costs. Physician reimbursement has already been agreed on, with LTNET committing to pay a fixed amount per physician work relative value unit (RVU). Thus, the primary matter at hand involves only Phase 4 hospital costs. To aid in the negotiations, Josh compiled the Phase 4 hospital costs of the 12 most recent liver transplant patients. These data are presented in Exhibit 9.1.

When Dr. Desai read the numbers, she was amazed. A total average cost of $119,805 for 19 days average length of stay (ALOS) translates to a per diem average cost of more than $6,000. She was sure that LTNET would not be willing to sign a contract that paid the hospital $120,000 (or more) to cover Phase 4 hospital costs. Thus, Dr. Desai suggested that Josh reexamine the cost structure to see if these costs could be reduced.

At first glance, it appeared to Josh that a large cost savings could be realized by merely reducing ALOS. For example, it appeared that Phase 4 hospital costs associated with a particular patient could be reduced by more than $12,000 by merely reducing ALOS by two days. However, further analysis revealed that the costs associated with Phase 4 are not a linear function of ALOS. Internal studies at the Center indicated that the first day of Phase 4 is usually the most costly while the last day is usually the least costly. Indeed, roughly 70 percent of Phase 4 costs occur in the first 24 hours of hospitalization.

When it appeared that it would be difficult to lower Phase 4 hospital costs, Josh decided to pursue a different strategy. He believed that economies of scale are present in liver transplants, and hence the marginal cost of each transplant is lower than the average cost. Thus, Josh proposed that the Phase 4 hospital reimbursement amount be based on marginal rather than total (full) costs.

Assume that you have been hired as a consultant to recommend a fixed reimbursement amount (the base rate) that should be proposed in the contract negotiations for Phase 4 hospital services. To help in the analysis, Josh has indicated that approximately 60 percent of nursing, ancillary, operating room, and laboratory costs are fixed. The remaining costs—radiology, drug, and other services—are predominantly variable.

Furthermore, current payers are reimbursing the hospital at roughly $140,000 for Phase 4 services.

The Center has sufficient capacity to handle about 30 more transplants before fixed costs would increase by a meaningful amount. If marginal volume exceeds 30 transplants, the best estimate is that fixed costs would increase somewhere between 15 and 25 percent.

In addition, you have been asked to recommend a method for handling outliers, including the threshold amount and additional reimbursement scheme. Other programs within the Center use two methods for outlier payments. One method is to charge an additional per diem amount based on a length-of-stay threshold. Alternatively, some percentage of costs above the threshold can be charged when a cost threshold is reached. (For more information on how Medicare treats outliers, go to www.cms.hhs.gov/mlngeninfo and then search "inpatient outliers.")

As you think about the problem at hand, several other issues come to mind. First, would it be useful to identify the underlying cost structure of the Phase 4 hospital services? (It might help in thinking about the relevant issues.) Second, should the hospital worry about a long-term pricing strategy, or is it sufficient to think only in terms of the first-year contract? Finally, if the price is set significantly lower than the average reimbursement amount paid by current payers, what impact would that have on future negotiations with those payers?

EXHIBIT 9.1
Cambridge Transplant Center: Phase 4 Hospital Costs (millions of dollars)

Patient	Age (years)	LOS (days)	Total Costs	Nursing Cost	Ancillary Cost	OR Cost	Lab Cost	Radiology Cost	Drug Cost	Other Costs
A	61	25	$141,092	$10,261	$65,416	$6,770	$13,712	$1,483	$20,992	$22,458
B	56	15	139,306	11,969	63,668	8,501	7,409	2,261	24,504	20,994
C	42	12	74,259	6,939	33,661	3,128	5,279	668	6,964	17,620
D	52	13	115,349	7,221	54,063	5,779	6,112	903	7,638	33,633
E	12	26	172,613	28,205	72,204	6,847	10,550	1,766	23,061	29,980
F	59	22	83,807	16,858	33,474	4,654	6,211	1,397	9,698	11,515
G	41	25	136,060	9,645	63,208	6,489	13,091	1,382	20,127	22,118
H	35	17	139,308	11,969	63,669	8,501	7,409	2,261	24,505	20,994
I	52	12	74,259	6,939	33,660	3,128	5,280	668	6,964	17,620
J	38	13	115,348	7,221	54,063	5,778	6,111	903	7,639	33,633
K	59	25	166,224	26,909	69,657	6,765	10,061	1,677	22,007	29,148
L	60	21	80,034	15,629	32,202	4,531	5,937	1,293	9,122	11,320
Average	47	19	$119,805	$13,314	$53,245	$5,906	$8,097	$1,389	$15,268	$22,586

LOS: length of stay; OR: operating room

DALLAS HEALTH NETWORK

ABC ANALYSIS

10

DALLAS HEALTH NETWORK (the Network), which consists of five medical group practices, is a subsidiary of not-for-profit Dallas Health System (the System). The Network includes both primary care and specialty physicians, with an emphasis on obstetrics/gynecology, eldercare, and pediatrics. Prior to the founding of the Network, the five practices operated independently.

The Network has three practice locations, each staffed with a mix of primary care and specialist physicians. Although the Network itself is only marginally profitable, it is an important contributor to System profitability because it generates a large amount of revenues for other System components from referrals for both inpatient admissions and inpatient and outpatient ancillary services. In fact, it has been estimated that each $1 of revenue generated within the Network leads to $8 of inpatient and ancillary revenues to the System. By limiting the amount of ancillary services provided at the three Network locations, patients are forced (or at least encouraged) to use other System facilities for such services.

Still, some ancillary services are best performed at the Network locations for one or more of the following reasons: lower costs, increased physician efficiency, or improved patient convenience and hence better CAHPS (Consumer Assessment of Healthcare Providers and Systems) scores. For example, one of the practice locations now has a diagnostic imaging capability. When the scanner was moved from another facility to the Network location, volume increased, costs

75

decreased, and both physician and patient satisfaction improved. (For more information on the CAHPS program, see www.cahps.ahrq.gov/ about.htm.)

The proposal now being considered by the Network is to provide ultrasound services at the Network locations. Preliminary analysis indicates that two approaches are most suitable. Alternative 1 involves the purchase of one ultrasound machine for each of the Network's three locations. Patients would schedule appointments, generally at the clinic they are using, during preset times on specified days of the week. Then, the full-time ultrasound technician would travel from one location to another to administer the tests as scheduled.

In Alternative 2, patient scheduling would be the same, but only one ultrasound machine would be purchased. It would be mounted in a van that the technician would drive to each of the three Network locations. Most of the operating costs of the two alternatives are identical, but Alternative 2 has the added cost of operating the van and setting up the machine after each move.

The two alternatives differ substantially in capital investment costs because Alternative 1 requires three ultrasound machines, at a cost of $100,000 each, while Alternative 2 requires only one. However, Alternative 2 requires a van, which with necessary modifications would cost $40,000. Thus, the capital costs for Alternative 1 total 3 x $100,000 = $300,000, while those for Alternative 2 amount to only $100,000 + $40,000 = $140,000.

Note, though, that because the two alternatives have different operating costs, a proper cost analysis of the two alternatives must include both capital investment and operating costs. The Network financial staff, which in reality is the System financial staff, considered several methods for estimating the operating costs of each alternative. After much discussion, the chief financial officer (CFO) decided that the activity based costing (ABC) method would be best. Furthermore, an ad hoc task force was assigned to perform the cost analysis.

To begin the ABC analysis, the task force had to develop the activities involved in the two alternatives. This was accomplished by conducting walk-throughs of the entire process from the standpoints of the patient, the ultrasound technician, and the billing and collections department. The results are shown in Exhibit 10.1. A review of the activities confirms that all except one—consisting of transportation, setup, and breakdown—are applicable to both alternatives.

The next step in the ABC process is to detail the costs associated with each activity. This step uses financial, operational, and volume data, along with the appropriate cost driver for each activity, to estimate resource consumption. Note that traditional costing, which often focuses on department-level costs, typically first deals with direct costs and then allocates indirect (overhead) costs proportionally according to a predetermined allocation rate. In ABC costing, the activities required to produce some service, including both direct and indirect, are estimated simultaneously. For example, Exhibit 10.1 contains activities that entail direct costs (such as technician time) and activities that entail indirect costs (such as billing and collection). Although the ABC method is more complex and hence costlier than the traditional method, it is the only way to accurately (more or less) estimate the costs of individual services.

Activity cost detail on a per procedure basis is contained in Exhibit 10.2. In essence, each activity is assigned a cost driver that is most highly correlated with the actual utilization of resources. Then, the number of driver units, along with the cost per unit, is estimated for each activity. The product of the number of units and the cost per unit gives the cost of each activity. Finally, the activity costs are summed to obtain the total per procedure cost.

Many of the activity costs cannot be estimated without an estimate of the number of ultrasounds that will be performed. The best estimate is that 50 procedures would be done each week, regardless of which alternative is chosen. Assuming the technician works 48 weeks per year, the annual volume estimate is 2,400 procedures. Of course, one factor that complicates the analysis is that a much greater total volume can be accommodated under Alternative 1, with three machines, than with Alternative 2, with only one machine. However, to keep the initial analysis manageable, the decision was made to assume the same annual volume regardless of the alternative chosen.

In addition to the costs mentioned thus far, some other costs are thought to be relevant to the decision. First, in addition to the obvious costs of purchasing and operating (primarily fuel expenses) the van, it is estimated that annual vehicle maintenance costs will run about $1,000. Furthermore, annual maintenance costs on each of the three machines under Alternative 1 are estimated at $1,000, while the annual maintenance costs for the single machine under Alternative 2 are estimated higher, at $1,500, because of added wear and tear. Also, the manufacturer of the ultrasound machines has indicated that a discount may be available if three machines, as opposed to only one, are purchased. The amount of the discount is somewhat uncertain, although 5 percent has been mentioned.

Finally, to have a rough estimate of total annual costs over the life of the equipment, it is necessary to make assumptions about the useful life of the ultrasound machines and the van. Although somewhat controversial, the decision was made to assume a five-year life for both the ultrasound machines and the van. Furthermore, the assumption was made that the value of these assets would be negligible at the end of five years.

Assume that you are the chairperson of the ad hoc task force. Your charge is to evaluate the two alternatives and to make a recommendation on which one to accept, assuming that revenues would be identical for the two alternatives and, hence, the decision can be made solely on the basis of costs. As part of the analysis, it will be necessary to estimate the costs of the two alternatives on a per procedure and an annual basis. In addition, any qualitative factors that are relevant to the decision must be considered before the recommendation is made.

To keep the analysis manageable, the task force was instructed to assume that operating costs remain constant over the useful life of the equipment. For comparative purposes, this assumption is not too egregious because the activities are roughly the same for both alternatives and, hence, inflation would have a somewhat neutral impact on the cost comparison.

In addition to the base case analysis, the System CFO has asked the task force to perform some sensitivity (scenario) analyses. First, he is concerned about the accuracy of the cost detail inputs. Although there is some confidence in many of the estimates, others are more arbitrary. Those activity cost inputs that are considered to be most uncertain are supplies cost per unit; billing and collection cost per unit; general administration cost per unit; and transportation, setup, and breakdown cost per unit. Thus, the task force has been asked to redo the analysis assuming that these inputs are higher than the base case values by 10 and 20 percent. Activity cost inputs less than the base case values could also be examined, but the critical issue here is not to underestimate the total costs involved in the two alternatives.

Second, and along the same lines, the task force was asked what would happen to the cost estimates if the useful life of the capital equipment was as short as three years or as long as seven years. Also, concern was expressed that the useful life of the equipment depended on the alternative chosen; that is, there would be less wear and tear under Alternative 1 than under Alternative 2. Finally, the task force was asked to assess the impact of a purchase discount—would the discount amount influence the ultimate decision?

Although you believe that it also would be very useful to perform a sensitivity analysis on the number of procedures, this task would require recalculation of the per unit cost inputs, an effort thought to be too time consuming to undertake at this point in the analysis.

1. Appointment scheduling
2. Patient check-in
3. Ultrasound testing
4. Patient check-out
5. Film processing
6. Film reading
7. Billing and collection
8. General administration
9. Transportation, setup, and breakdown (Alternative 2 only)

EXHIBIT 10.1
Dallas Health Network:
Activities Associated
with Alternatives 1 and 2

EXHIBIT 10.2
Dallas Health Network:
Activity Cost Detail

Activity	Cost Driver	Volume	Cost per Unit
Appointment scheduling	Receptionist time	3 minutes	$ 0.20
Patient check-in	Receptionist time	5 minutes	0.20
Ultrasound testing	Technician time	30 minutes	0.40
	Physician time	1.5 minutes	3.00
	Supplies	per procedure	9.00
Patient check-out	Receptionist time	5 minutes	0.20
Film processing	Technician time	10 minutes	0.40
Film reading	Contract terms	per procedure	40.00
Billing and collection	Overhead costs	per procedure	6.80
General administration	Overhead costs	per procedure	1.25
Transportation, setup, and breakdown	Technician time	18 minutes	1.00

Notes: 1. Physician time for testing (15 minutes) is needed for one of every ten patients.
   2. Supplies consist of linen, probe cover, gel, film, and print paper.
   3. There are no radiologists in the Network. Films will be read by the Hospital's
       radiologists at a contract fee of $40 per procedure.
   4. Billing and collection costs are based on an average cost per medical services bill.
   5. General administration costs are based on an estimate of facilities and other
       administrative costs.
   6. Transportation, setup, and breakdown are based on ten procedures per day and
       include vehicle operating costs, excluding maintenance.

ORLANDO FAMILY PHYSICIANS

11

PAY FOR
PERFORMANCE

ORLANDO FAMILY PHYSICIANS is a medical group practice located in Orlando, Maine. The practice has four family practice physicians and a medical support staff consisting of a practice manager, two receptionists, four nurses, two medical assistants, two billing clerks, and one laboratory technician. Data relevant to the practice are shown in Exhibits 11.1 through 11.3.

The practice is organized as a partnership, with each physician having an equal share. Although the practice manager has the authority to make the day-to-day business decisions, all strategic decisions regarding the management of the practice are made jointly by the partners. In addition, the practice uses a local CPA (certified public accountant) to prepare and file its taxes and to act as a financial adviser when needed.

The current policy of the practice is to provide equal compensation to the physicians. Last year, each physician was paid the same monthly salary ($12,500) and, at the end of the year, profits of the practice that were not needed for reinvestment in new assets were divided equally among the partners ($30,000 each). Although this policy of "equal pay for equal work" has been in place since the practice was founded in 1996, there is growing discontent among the partners regarding this compensation system. Not surprisingly, each of the physicians believes that he or she is working harder than the others and hence should receive greater compensation. In addition, the physicians have recognized that it is important to start putting away some profits to pay for new medical equipment that will replace aging items and expand the range of services offered.

A recent survey by the Medical Group Management Association indicated that less than 10 percent of group practice family physicians are compensated on a straight salary basis, while the majority are compensated on the basis of productivity. Of those compensated on the basis of productivity measures, about half are paid solely on productivity and half receive a base salary plus a "bonus" component based either on productivity exclusively or on productivity plus other measures. (For more information on the Medical Group Management Association, see www.mgma.com.)

In an effort to both reward those physicians who are truly "working harder" and create the incentive for all physicians to be as productive as possible, the partners directed the practice manager to assess the current compensation system and to recommend any changes that would improve the system.

Assume that you are the practice manager of Orlando Family Physicians. As a start, you scheduled a meeting with the partners to gain some initial guidance. At this meeting, the partners agreed that any proposed system must have the following five characteristics:

1. The system must be **trusted.** Physicians must trust not only the data used but also the integrity and competency of the individuals who administer the system. The compensation model itself may be sound, but a lack of faith in either the data or the administration of the system will lead to a lack of confidence in the entire system.
2. The system must be clearly **understood.** In the search for the perfect system, it is all too easy to create a model that is overly complex, and hence the links between pay and performance cannot be easily identified. If the physicians cannot easily identify what performance is necessary to increase pay, the system will not have the desired results.
3. The system must be perceived to be **equitable.** If the physicians do not believe that the system is fair—that is, those physicians who contribute more are paid more—it is doomed to failure.
4. The system must create the proper **incentives.** A fundamental objective of any compensation plan is to maintain the financial viability of the organization.

Thus, the model must create incentives that promote behavior that contributes to the success of the group. Furthermore, the incentives offered must be large enough to encourage physicians to change behavior.

5. The system must be **affordable.** The costs of implementing and administering the system must be reasonable. Furthermore, the total amount of incentive compensation paid must not impair the ability of the practice to cover its operating costs, replace existing assets, or acquire new assets.

There was general agreement among the physicians that the compensation system should be base salary plus some form of pay for performance. For example, each physician might receive a base salary of $6,000 per month and the remaining compensation would be based on some measure(s) of performance.

Even with this agreement, the task of making recommendations for change in the physician compensation system seemed daunting. After all, there are many systems available, each with its own strengths and weaknesses. To gain a better appreciation of the possible choices, you downloaded from the Internet several articles about pay for performance and met with Jennifer Wong, the group's accountant, to learn about the alternative systems being used at other practices. After several meetings with Jennifer, you conclude that several potential measures might be appropriate for Orlando's pay-for-performance plan.

Productivity measures:
- *Number of patient visits.* This measure is a simple count of the annual number of patient visits for a physician, regardless of the time per visit or type of patient. More patient visits indicate higher physician productivity.
- *Work relative value units (RVUs).* Jennifer consulted with another group practice that uses RVUs to measure productivity. RVUs form the basis of physician compensation for Medicare services. Under this system, each physician service has three relative value components: (1) physician work, (2) practice expense, and (3) malpractice expense. More work RVUs indicate higher productivity.

- *Professional procedures.* This measure is a simple count of the annual number of procedure codes (such as injections), regardless of the time per procedure, type of procedure, or reimbursement amount. More professional procedures indicate higher productivity.

Financial measures:
- *Gross charges.* This measure is the total gross charges generated by a physician during the year (discounts, allowances, and costs are ignored). Gross charges are easily identified from the current billing system used by the practice. More gross charges indicate higher physician financial performance.
- *Net collections.* This measure is the total collected revenue generated by a physician during the year (gross charges minus discounts and allowances; again, costs are ignored). Net collections are also easily identified from the current billing system used by the practice. More net collections indicate higher financial performance.
- *Net income.* This measure is the total net income (before physician compensation) generated by a physician during the year. As stated above, gross charges and net collections are easily identified from the current billing system used by the practice. However, this measure requires allocation of practice costs to individual physicians. With limited data at hand, one possible solution is to divide the total costs of the practice into fixed and variable components and then allocate the fixed component equally to all four physicians and allocate the variable component on the basis of some measure of resource utilization, such as professional procedures. Higher net income indicates higher financial performance.

Quality measures:
- *Average patient satisfaction.* This measure is an average of the patient satisfaction scores for a physician. Higher patient satisfaction scores indicate higher physician quality.

- *Blood pressure control.* This measure indicates whether or not a physician met a target for blood pressure control among the patients seen during the year. The Centers for Medicare & Medicaid Services (CMS) is currently sponsoring the Physician Group Practice (PGP) Demonstration (see www.cms.hhs. gov/DemoProjectsEvalRpts/downloads/PGP_Demo_Design.pdf). Participating physicians are eligible to earn separate quality payments if they meet performance targets on a variety of quality measures. Blood pressure control is one of the quality measures that apply to all Medicare beneficiaries that meet age and sex criteria. Attaining the target indicates higher quality.
- *Breast cancer screening.* This is another PGP Demonstration quality measure that applies to all Medicare beneficiaries that meet age and sex criteria. Attaining the target indicates higher quality.

Of course, any combination of the above measures could also be used, so a wide variety of solutions is possible.

Armed with the above information, you held another meeting with the partners and Jennifer to gain some additional insights into their views regarding physician compensation. The meeting had three agenda items: (1) Should pay for performance be based on productivity, financial performance, and/or quality? (2) What total dollar amount should be allocated to performance pay versus base salary? (3) What amount of net income (after physician compensation) should the group target?

At the beginning of the meeting, all agreed that the physicians who contribute most to the practice should receive the highest compensation. However, it soon became clear that there was no agreement on how to define "contribute most." For example, one physician stated that work effort is the most meaningful measure. "Let's just use the number of patient visits—it's simple, and we all agree that more visits require more work," he argued. But this was challenged by another physician, who stated that many of her patients were elderly and chronically ill who require much more time per visit than do younger, healthier patients. Work RVUs would be another basis of measuring productivity, but the physicians weren't sure about using data from a billing system for such a purpose. Another physician argued that the real money is in procedures. Historically, physicians have been paid relatively well for diagnostic and treatment procedures, and group practices that do a lot of procedures have done well financially. Therefore, it made sense to consider rewarding those physicians who performed higher numbers of professional procedures. But another physician was uncomfortable with rewarding such a narrow part of clinical practice. "Besides," he said, "I am getting older and don't do as many procedures as I once did."

Next, the discussion turned to financial performance measures. Although one physician strongly believed that gross charges were the best measure, another countered that (1) gross charges do not reflect reimbursement amounts and (2) gross charges generated at the expense of high costs do not help the group much financially. Jennifer jumped in at that point, saying that the strength of the net income measure is that physicians are held responsible for both revenues and costs. Thus, physicians would have the incentive to be more productive (generate more revenues) while reducing the costs associated with operating the practice. However, the cost allocation required for calculation of net income can only be roughly estimated, so it will be difficult to convince the physicians that the allocation has true economic meaning.

Performance pay based on quality was the last item discussed. One physician stated that there is too much emphasis on money. If the physicians do not provide high-quality medical care and keep their patients happy, there will be no patients and hence no revenues. Thus, she argued, "Patient satisfaction is just as important as revenue generation." In addition to the patient satisfaction issue, one partner noted that Orlando physicians provide care to many Medicare beneficiaries. "It's important to gain experience with the pay-for-quality approach that CMS is supporting," he argued. However, the reaction to this comment was mixed. Two partners thought the whole idea of rewarding physicians for practicing good medicine was ludicrous. One commented that the profession is in a sad state of affairs if physicians have to be paid extra to do what is right. On the other hand, another partner stated that if this were the trend among payers, it might be wise to consider building similar quality guidelines into Orlando's compensation system.

At the end of the discussion on Agenda Item 1, one physician stated, "It's clear we don't agree on how to measure performance, so why don't we just use all of the measures? Then everybody will be happy." The thought of using all of the measures made you shudder because of the complexity of interpreting the results and the administrative burden that would be required.

Then, the meeting turned to Agenda Item 2: the actual amount to be allocated to performance pay. One physician suggested that because there was no agreement on how to measure performance, most compensation should be base salary and only a small amount should be allocated for performance pay—say, $10,000 per physician. This brought a chorus of "why bother" from the other physicians. "This isn't enough of an incentive for anything—after all, we spend more than that on lattes," one joked. In contrast, another physician stated, "I'd prefer to base all of our compensation on performance; who can argue with productivity, financial performance, and quality?" After a prolonged discussion, the only agreement was that the dollar amount allocated to performance pay should be enough to make physicians pay attention to it but less than the amount allocated for base salary.

Agenda Item 3 revolved around the target net income (after physician compensation). In contrast to their dissension on the other agenda items, all of the physicians readily agreed that the net income after physician compensation of the practice had to be at least $70,000 to pay for new medical equipment that the practice requires.

At the end of the meeting, you could tell that the job would not be an easy one. None of the approaches initially identified could be ruled out. Furthermore, there was only broad direction on the dollar amount to be allocated for performance pay. Your major hurdle will be to develop a system that would be supported by all four partners. Thus, the ability to "sell" the system to the partners is just as important as the system itself.

To ensure an orderly approach to the assignment, you decide to (1) use the historical allocation between base salary and performance pay as a starting point, (2) assess the sensitivity of physician pay to the various performance measures, and (3) recommend the system that you believe is best for Orlando Family Physicians. Finally, you recognize that the merits of alternative compensation systems are influenced somewhat by the nature of the practice's revenue stream (reimbursement). Almost half of the practice's revenues come from Medicare and Medicaid, with the remainder coming from commercial insurers, including managed care plans. Although some of the managed care plans were using capitated payment systems several years ago, all of the practice's payers now use fee-for-service methodologies.

EXHIBIT 11.1
Orlando Family
Physicians: Historical
Support Staff Salaries

	Number of Employees	Total Compensation
Practice manager	1	$ 75,168
Receptionists	2	48,652
Nurses	4	175,264
Medical assistants	2	52,615
Billing clerks	2	62,165
Laboratory technician	1	46,788
Other staffing costs		61,736
Total		$522,388

Note: Other staffing costs include accounting and other fees for outsourced services.

Gross charges	$2,242,648
Net collections	$1,747,059
Practice expenses:	
Support staff salaries	$ 522,388
Facilities cost	298,351
Supplies cost	136,257
Total practice expenses	$ 956,996
Net income before physician compensation	$ 790,063
Physician compensation:	
Base salaries	$ 600,000
Bonus	120,000
Total physician compensation	$ 720,000
Net income after physician compensation	$ 70,063

EXHIBIT 11.2
Orlando Family
Physicians: Historical
Financial Data

	Physician Identifier				
	A	B	C	D	Total
Patient visits	4,023	3,567	3,966	4,244	15,800
Number of RVUs	4,667	5,055	5,475	4,967	20,164
Professional procedures	6,255	6,972	7,287	6,742	27,256
Gross charges	$527,820	$535,841	$602,675	$567,312	$2,242,648
Net collections	$422,256	$401,881	$421,872	$501,050	$1,747,059
Average patient satisfaction score	89	80	87	94	
Blood pressure control target met?	Yes	Yes	Yes	No	
Breast cancer screening target met?	No	Yes	No	No	

RVUs: relative value units

Notes: 1. The RVUs listed are work RVUs, which are only one of the three components used in Medicare physician reimbursement.
2. Over the past five years, the average annual amount reinvested in the practice was $65,000.
3. Patient satisfaction scores are measured using a 100-point scale.

EXHIBIT 11.3
Orlando Family
Physicians: Historical
Physician Data

Financial Management Basics

GULF SHORES SURGERY CENTERS

TIME VALUE ANALYSIS

12

GARY HUDSON was born and raised in Pensacola, Florida. He obtained his bachelor's degree in business from Florida State University, where he enrolled in the NROTC (Naval Reserve Officers Training Corps) program. After graduation, he received a commission in the US Marine Corps. Following his release from active duty, Gary used his GI Bill benefits to obtain a master's degree in health services administration from the University of Florida. His first job in healthcare was as a special projects coordinator/financial analyst at a large Miami hospital. He enjoyed his work there, but his ultimate goal was to return to Pensacola as the manager of a smaller healthcare business, where he would have more responsibility and authority. After five years in Miami, Gary became the chief operating and financial officer of Gulf Shores Surgery Centers, an investor-owned chain of ambulatory surgery centers with six locations in Florida's Panhandle.

Immediately after assuming his new position, Gary found himself facing several decisions. First, Gary had to select a bank or banks to meet the financial needs of Gulf Shores. He has approached two local banks—Sun Trust and BankSouth—about the interest rates they offer on a savings account and a certificate of deposit (CD) as well as the rate charged on a term loan (Exhibit 12.1).

Second, a wealthy patient was so impressed with the care she received at Gulf Shores that she decided to make a series of donations to the facility. She will donate $75,000 a year for the first six years ($t = 1$ through $t = 6$, where $t = $ time) and $150,000 annually for the following six years ($t = 7$ through $t = 12$). The first deposit will be made a

93

year from today. In addition, she has just written a check for $250,000, which Gary will invest immediately (t = 0). Gary will invest all of the donations in a CD as they become available. CDs are generally offered in maturities of from six months to ten years, and interest can be handled in one of two ways: the investor (buyer) can receive periodic interest payments, or the interest can automatically be reinvested in the CD. In the latter case, the buyer receives no interest during the life of the CD but receives the accumulated interest plus the principal amount at maturity. Because the goal of this investment is to accumulate funds for future use, as opposed to generating current income, all interest earned on the CD would be reinvested.

Third, Gulf Shores may launch substantial building renovations. In this circumstance, it would be forced to borrow $250,000 from a bank. Gary is considering two options for a term loan:

1. A five-year term loan that would be repaid in equal annual installments, with the first payment due at the end of Year 1. Gary hopes to pay off the loan early—at the end of Year 3.
2. A seven-year loan that would be repaid in annual installments of differing amounts, with the first payment due at the end of Year 1. For the first three years of the loan, the annual installment would be projected cash surpluses ($25,000 at the end of Year 1, $50,000 at the end of Year 2, and $75,000 at the end of Year 3). For the final four years of the loan, the annual installment would be a fixed but currently unspecified cash flow, X, at the end of each year from Year 4 through Year 7.

Finally, Gulf Shores has a board-designated building fund to pay for projected facility renovations starting in eight years and lasting for four years (at t = 8, 9, 10, and 11). Current building renovation costs are estimated to be $14,500,000 a year, but they are expected to increase at a rate of 3.5 percent a year. So far, Gulf Shores has accumulated $15,000,000 (at t = 0). Gary's long-run financial plan is to add $5,000,000 in each of the next four years (at t = 1, 2, 3, and 4). Then, he plans to make equal annual contributions in each of the following three years (t = 5, 6, and 7).

All of the decisions Gary faces involve time value analysis.

Bank	Product	Compounding	Nominal Interest Rate
Sun Trust	Savings account	Daily	4.00%
	Certificate of deposit	Monthly	6.00%
	Term loan	Quarterly	8.00%
BankSouth	Savings account	Weekly	4.10%
	Certificate of deposit	Annually	6.10%
	Term loan	Semiannually	8.06%

EXHIBIT 12.1
Interest Rates on Three Financial Products

MID-ATLANTIC
SPECIALTY, INC.

FINANCIAL RISK

13

MID-ATLANTIC SPECIALTY, INC. (MSI) is a not-for-profit corporation formed by physicians in the College of Medicine at Mid-Atlantic University. MSI, with more than 600 physicians, provides the medical staff for University Hospital. In addition, MSI staffs and administers a network of 25 ambulatory care clinics and centers at ten locations within 50 miles of the hospital. In 2013, MSI generated over $500 million in revenues from about 40,000 inpatient stays and 750,000 outpatient visits.

More than 70 percent of MSI's revenues currently come from inpatient stays, but this percentage has been declining; by 2018, over half of MSI's revenues are expected to stem from outpatient services. As improvements are made in technology and as third-party payers continue to pressure providers to cut costs, more and more inpatient services will be converted to outpatient and home care. For example, in 2003, 80 percent of MSI's ophthalmological surgeries took place in University Hospital, whereas in 2013, 80 percent were performed in outpatient settings.

Although MSI has traditionally provided only specialty services, in 2012 it instituted a "personal physician services" program, in which patients can receive both primary and specialty care from College of Medicine physicians. This was the first step in MSI's drive to develop an integrated delivery system, which offers a full range of patient services. Now that the system is in place, MSI is contracting with managed care plans to provide virtually all physician services required locally by plan members. Furthermore, MSI is examining the feasibility of contracting

97

directly with employers, and hence bypassing managed care plans, but no decision has yet been made. Indeed, state insurance industry representatives expressed opposition to the idea when MSI first announced the possibility of direct contracting. The insurance industry position is that direct contracting with employers to provide a complete healthcare benefit package is an insurance function, which can be undertaken only by licensed insurance plans.

As part of its continuing education program, MSI holds monthly "nonclinical grand rounds" for its physicians, in which various staff members and outside specialists conduct seminars on nonclinical topics of interest. As part of this series, Chris Johnson, MSI's chief financial officer, has been invited to conduct two sessions on the financial risk inherent in integrated delivery systems. His main concern is that physicians, although very sophisticated in clinical matters, have a limited understanding of basic financial risk concepts and will not appreciate the financial issues involved in integrated delivery systems without first gaining an understanding of financial risk fundamentals. Thus, he plans to devote the entire first session to basic concepts.

In preparation for the seminar, Chris estimated the one-year return distributions for the five investments shown in Exhibit 13.1. To create the table, he first hypothesized that there could be five possible economic states for the coming year, ranging from poor to excellent. Next, he estimated the one-year returns on each investment under each state. The five investments are (1) T-bills, (2) real asset investment Project A, (3) real asset investment Project B, (4) an index fund designed to proxy the returns on the Standard & Poor's (S&P) 500 stock index, and (5) an equity investment in MSI itself. T-bills are short-term (one-year or less maturity) US Treasury debt securities, Project A is a proposed sports medicine clinic, and Project B is a Medicaid-funded project for providing family health services to an underserved area. Chris developed the returns for Projects A and B and for MSI as a whole by assessing the impact of each economic state on healthcare utilization and reimbursement patterns. Finally, Chris assembled historical return distributions on the five investments shown in Exhibit 13.2. The historical returns for an existing sports medicine clinic and family health service were used for Projects A and B.

This information is the starting point for Chris to prepare his presentation on analysis of stand-alone, corporate, and market risk.

State of the Economy	Probability	Investment				
		1-Year T-Bill	Project A	Project B	S&P 500 Fund	Equity in MSI
Poor	0.1	7%	–8%	18%	–15%	0%
Below average	0.2	7%	2%	23%	0%	5%
Average	0.4	7%	14%	7%	15%	10%
Above average	0.2	7%	25%	–3%	30%	15%
Excellent	0.1	7%	33%	2%	45%	20%

EXHIBIT 13.1
Mid-Atlantic Specialty, Inc.: Estimated One-Year Return Distributions on Five Investments

	1-Year T-Bill	Project A	Project B	S&P 500 Fund	Equity in MSI
Year 1	7%	–8%	18%	–15%	0%
Year 2	7%	2%	23%	0%	5%
Year 3	7%	14%	7%	15%	10%
Year 4	7%	25%	–3%	30%	15%
Year 5	7%	33%	2%	45%	20%

EXHIBIT 13.2
Mid-Atlantic Specialty, Inc.: Historical Return Distributions on Five Investments

Note: These return distributions are fictitious and not meant to describe actual market conditions at the time you work this case.

PACIFIC HEALTHCARE (A)
BOND VALUATION

14

PACIFIC HEALTHCARE IS an investor-owned hospital chain that owns and operates nine hospitals in Washington, Oregon, and Northern California. Marcia Long, a recent graduate of a prominent health administration program, has just been hired by Washington Medical Center, Pacific's largest hospital. Like all new management personnel, Marcia must undergo three months of intensive indoctrination at the system level before joining the hospital.

Marcia began her indoctrination in January 2014. Her first assignment at Pacific was to review its latest annual report. This was a stroke of luck for Marcia because her father owned several bonds issued by Pacific, and Marcia was especially interested in whether or not her father had made a good investment. To glean more information about the bonds, Marcia examined Note E to Pacific's consolidated financial statements, which lists the company's long-term debt obligations, including its first mortgage bonds, installment contracts, and term loans. Exhibit 14.1 contains information on four of the first-mortgage bonds listed in Pacific's annual report. All four bonds pay interest semiannually. (For more information on bond ratings, see Standard & Poor's website at www.standardpoor.com or the Moody's Investors Service website at http://moodys.com.)

Pacific's chief financial officer, Hugo Welsh, found out about Marcia's interest in the firm's debt financing. "Because you are so interested in our financial structure," he said, "I want you to do the bond valuation and make a presentation to our executive committee."

Hugo then asked Marcia to perform the calculations required to complete Exhibit 14.2 and to think about some of the questions that members of the committee might ask her about the numbers.

EXHIBIT 14.1
Pacific Healthcare:
Long-Term Bonds

Face Amount	Current Price	Par Value	Coupon Rate	Maturity Date	Years to Maturity	Bond Rating
$ 48,000,000	$ 800.00	$1,000	4.50%	12/31/2018	5	A+
$ 32,000,000	$ 865.49	$1,000	8.25%	12/31/2028	15	A+
$100,000,000	$1,220.00	$1,000	12.625%	12/31/2038	25	A+
$ 64,000,000	$ 747.48	$1,000	7.375%	12/31/2038	25	A+

EXHIBIT 14.2
Pacific Healthcare:
Long-Term Bond Stated
(Nominal) Yields

Face Amount	Annual YTM	2014 Coupon Payments	2014 Current Yield	1/1/2015 Expected Price	2014 Capital Gain Yield	2014 Total Yield
$ 48,000,000						
$ 32,000,000						
$100,000,000						
$ 64,000,000						

YTM: yield to maturity

PACIFIC HEALTHCARE (B)
STOCK VALUATION

15

PACIFIC HEALTHCARE IS an investor-owned hospital chain that owns and operates nine hospitals in Washington, Oregon, and Northern California. Marcia Long, a recent graduate of a prominent health services administration program, has just been hired by Washington Medical Center, Pacific's largest hospital. Like all new management personnel, Marcia must undergo three months of intensive indoctrination at the system level before joining the hospital.

In Case 14, Marcia conducted an analysis of the firm's bonds and presented her findings to the company's executive committee. Pacific's chief financial officer, Hugo Welsh, was very impressed with the quality of Marcia's presentation. Furthermore, the other members of the committee stated that they learned a great deal about debt financing from Marcia's presentation and would like to see a similar presentation on equity financing. Because Marcia would be leaving corporate headquarters to start her hospital assignment in less than four weeks, Hugo immediately assigned her the task of analyzing the firm's equity situation and preparing another presentation for the executive committee.

Marcia began by reexamining the firm's annual report to get some basic financial data. Then, she searched Yahoo! Finance (http://finance.yahoo.com), CNNMoney (http://money.cnn.com/), Bloomberg (www.bloomberg.com/), and MSN Money (http://money.msn.com/) for current market data as well as analysts' forecasts for Pacific Healthcare and the market. She discovered that the stock of Pacific Healthcare is currently (on December 31, 2013) selling for $8 per share, its current dividend is $0.480 per share (paid on December 31, 2013), and its

103

beta coefficient is 1.2. Marcia also learned that the yield on long-term Treasury bonds is 5.0 percent and that a market return of 11 percent is expected. Most analysts forecast that Pacific will grow about 10 percent per year for the next five years (2014–2018) and 4 percent per year thereafter (2019 and beyond). Based on these growth forecasts, Marcia assembled the forecast dividends per share, as shown in Exhibit 15.1.

As before, Hugo did not want Marcia to go off on a tangent, so he told her that he was primarily interested in the current value of Pacific Healthcare's stock and whether it is under- or overvalued, the expected stock price over the next five years, and the expected dividend yield and capital gains yield over the next five years. He also suggested that Marcia think about some of the questions that members of the committee might ask her about the numbers.

EXHIBIT 15.1
Pacific Healthcare: Historical and Forecast Dividends per Share

	Year	Dividends per Share
Historical	2008	$0.215
	2009	$0.324
	2010	$0.353
	2011	$0.362
	2012	$0.391
	2013	$0.480
Forecast	2014	$0.528
	2015	$0.581
	2016	$0.639
	2017	$0.703
	2018	$0.773
	2019	$0.804
	2020	$0.836

Capital
Acquisition

SENIOR CARE ENTERPRISES

BOND REFUNDING

16

Senior Care Enterprises is a leading provider of post-acute healthcare. It is a for-profit corporation that operates more than 500 skilled nursing facilities, 30 assisted living centers, 150 outpatient rehabilitation therapy clinics, and 50 hospice and home care centers. Aram Catalan, the financial vice president of Senior Care Enterprises, is reviewing the minutes of the company's final 2009 board of directors meeting. The major topic discussed at the meeting was whether Senior Care should refund any of its currently outstanding bond issues. Of particular interest is a $100 million, 30-year bond issue sold approximately five years ago carrying an 8.0 percent coupon rate. Several of the board members had taken markedly different positions on the question, and, at the conclusion of the meeting, the chair of the board asked Aram to prepare a report analyzing the alternative points of view. (For more information on bonds, see the Investing in Bonds website at www.investingin bonds.com or the BondsOnline website at www.bondsonline.com.)

The bonds in question, which are rated single-A, were issued in January 2009 when interest rates were higher than they are today. Issuing the bonds at the time was necessary because Senior Care needed the capital to expand its rehabilitation services business line. Now, almost five years later, with lower rates, Senior Care can sell A-rated bonds that carry a lower interest rate than that set on the 2009 issue.

Because Aram wanted to have flexibility regarding when the 2009 issue could be retired, he had insisted that the bonds be made callable after five years. (If the bonds had not been callable, Senior Care Enterprises would have had to pay an interest rate of only 7.3 percent,

70 basis points less than the actual 8.0 percent coupon rate. If the bonds had been immediately callable, rather than having a deferred call, the coupon rate would have had to be pegged at 8.2 percent.) The bonds can be called on January 1, 2014 (the end of Year 5), but an initial call premium of one year's interest payment—$80 per $1,000 par value bond—would have to be paid. This premium declines by 8.0% ÷ 25 = 0.32 percentage points, or $3.20, each year. Thus, if the bonds were called on January 1, 2019 (the end of Year 10), the call premium would be (80% ÷ 25) × 20 = 6.4%, or $64, where 20 represents the number of years remaining to maturity. The flotation costs on this issue amounted to 1.5 percent of the face amount, or $1,500,000. Senior Care's federal-plus-state tax rate is 40 percent.

Aram estimates that Senior Care currently could sell a new issue of 25-year A-rated bonds at an interest rate of 7.0 percent. The call of the old and sale of the new bonds could take place five to seven weeks after the decision to refund has been made; this time is required to give legal notice to bondholders and arrange the financing needed to redeem the current issue. The flotation cost of the refunding issue would be 1 percent of the new issue's face amount, and funds from the new issue would be available from the underwriters the day they were needed to pay off the old bonds. Aram had proposed at the last directors' meeting that the company call the 8.0 percent bonds at the first opportunity and replace them with a new, lower coupon-rate issue. Although the refunding cost would be substantial, he believed the interest savings of 100 basis points per year for 25 years on a $100 million issue would be well worth the cost. Aram had not anticipated adverse reactions from any of the board members; however, three of them voiced strong reservations about his refunding proposal.

The first was Pamela Mathias, a long-term member of Senior Care's board and chair of Mathias & Company, an investment banking house that caters primarily to institutional clients such as insurance companies and pension funds. Pamela argued that calling the bonds for refunding would not be well received by the major institutions that hold Senior Care's outstanding bonds. According to Pamela, the institutional investors who hold the bonds purchased them on the expectation of receiving the 8.0 percent interest rate for at least ten years, and these investors would be very unhappy if a call occurred after only five years. Because most of the leading institutions hold some of Senior Care's bonds and because the firm typically sells new bonds to finance its growth every four or five years, it would be most unfortunate if institutional investors developed a feeling of ill will toward the company.

A second director, Vincent Marchiano, who is a relatively new member of the board and president of a local bank, also opposed the call, but for an entirely different reason. Vincent believed that the decline in interest rates was not yet over. He said a study by his bank suggested that the long-term interest rate on A-rated corporate bonds might fall to 6.0 percent next year. Under questioning from the other board members, however, Vincent admitted that the interest rate decline could in fact be over and that interest rates might begin to move back up again. When pressed, Vincent produced the following probability distribution that the bank's economists had developed for interest rates on A-rated corporate bonds one year from now (January 1, 2015):

Probability	Interest Rate on A-Rated Corporate Bonds
0.1	4%
0.2	5%
0.4	6%
0.2	7%
0.1	8%

The board agreed that any analysis of the impact of prospective interest rates on the refunding decision would assume that Senior Care would issue a 24-year bond if the refunding occurred one year hence.

The third director who opposed the call, Kim Mitchell, had lots of questions and wanted to fully understand all of the risks and returns before making a decision. She noted that interest rates had been quite volatile lately and that if rates rose before the new issue could be sold, but after the firm had committed to the refunding, the refunding would be a disaster. Therefore, she wondered how much interest rates could increase before Senior Care lost on the refunding. Indeed, the sensitivity of the refunding net present value to current interest rate levels would be a valuable tool in making the refunding decision. Another issue that Kim thought was of consequence to the refunding decision was tax rates. Senior Care's marginal tax rate could fall from its current value of 40 percent. Understanding the relationship between the attractiveness of refunding and the corporation's tax rate would be useful. Such an analysis could also show if the refunding decision is affected by ownership (for-profit versus not-for-profit) status.

As Aram's assistant, you have been asked to perform the bond refunding analysis and to report your conclusions and recommendations at the next executive committee meeting. With the model at hand, you begin your work, noting that, for ease of calculation, the model assumes annual coupons.

SEATTLE
CANCER CENTER
LEASING DECISIONS

17

SEATTLE CANCER CENTER (the Center) is a nationally known not-for-profit inpatient and outpatient facility dedicated to the prevention and treatment of cancer. Specific treatment services include surgery, chemotherapy, bone marrow transplantation, radiation therapy, and photodynamic therapy.

For the past ten years, the Center has been working diligently to perfect noninvasive brain surgery techniques. One technique, Gamma Knife radiosurgery, was developed in the 1950s and 1960s by Dr. Lars Leksell, a prominent Swedish neurosurgeon. The first patient treatment site was opened in 1968 in Stockholm, while the first site in the United States was established in Pittsburgh in 1977.

The Gamma Knife uses 201 separate radiation sources to treat certain brain cancers. Each radiation beam is quite weak and hence does not damage normal brain tissue, but when the separate beams are focused on a single point by a collimator helmet, the Gamma Knife delivers a dosage sufficient to be highly effective. The Gamma Knife is especially useful in the treatment of arteriovenous malformations, but it can also be used to treat certain types of benign tumors and even some small malignant lesions. The primary clinical benefit of the Gamma Knife is the significant reduction in the risk associated with traditional surgical procedures, in which the morbidity and mortality rates are substantial, especially for patients with deep lesions. In addition to treating cancer, the Gamma Knife can be used to treat functional disorders such as Parkinson's disease tremors and the pain that results from trigeminal neuralgia. (For more information about the Gamma Knife, including

111

an informative video on Gamma Knife surgery, see the manufacturer's website at http://gammaknife.org.)

The procedure calls for a team approach, including a neurosurgeon, radiation physicist, radiologist, and radiation therapist. The neurosurgeon selects the patients appropriate for the procedure and performs the stereotactic process required to localize the target area. The radiation physicist works with a computer program to compute the appropriate dosimetry, while the radiologist performs a CT (computed tomography) scan, an MRI (magnetic resonance imaging) scan, an angiogram, or a combination of the three to help the neurosurgeon localize the lesion.

The dosimetry calculations are especially complex. Because differing thicknesses of skull and brain will attenuate the beams in varying amounts, the amount of radiation applied is highly dependent on where the lesion is located and the size and shape of the patient's skull. The actual application of the radiation takes between 20 minutes and 2 hours, and the patient is generally released after only a short period of observation.

The Center plans to acquire a new Gamma Knife to replace its current model. The equipment has an invoice price of $3 million, including delivery and installation charges, and it falls into the MACRS (modified accelerated cost recovery system) five-year class, with current allowances of 0.20, 0.32, 0.19, 0.12, 0.11, and 0.06 in Years 1 through 6, respectively. The manufacturer of the equipment will provide a maintenance contract for $100,000 per year, payable at the beginning of each year, if the Center buys the equipment. Furthermore, the purchase could be financed by a four-year, simple-interest, conventional (taxable) bank note that would carry an interest rate of 8 percent.

Regardless of whether the equipment is purchased or leased, the Center's managers do not think the new Gamma Knife will be used for more than four years, at which time the Center plans to open a new radiation therapy facility. Land on which to construct a larger facility has already been acquired, and the building should be ready for occupancy at that time. The new facility is designed to enable the Center to use several new radiosurgery procedures. Thus, the Gamma Knife replacement is viewed as a "bridge," to serve only until the new facility is ready. The expected physical life of the equipment is ten years, but medical equipment of this nature is subject to unpredictable technological obsolescence.

After considerable debate among the Center's managers, they concluded that there is a 25 percent probability that the residual (salvage) value after four years will be $500,000; a 50 percent probability that it will be $1 million; and a 25 percent probability that it will be $2 million, which makes the residual value quite risky. Because the residual value is judged to have high risk, a 5 percentage point risk adjustment will be added to the base discount rate used on the other lease-analysis flows to obtain the appropriate rate for the residual value flows.

GB Financing (GBF), a leasing company that is partially owned by the manufacturer, has presented an initial offer to the Center to lease the equipment for annual payments of $675,000, with the first payment due on delivery and installation and subsequent payments due at the beginning of each succeeding year of the four-year lease term. This rental price includes a service contract under which the equipment would be maintained in good working order. GBF would buy the equipment from the manufacturer under the same terms that were offered to the Center, and GBF would have to enter into a maintenance contract with the manufacturer for $100,000 per year. (For more information on leasing healthcare equipment, see the GE Capital Healthcare Financial Services website at www.gehealthcarefinance.com.)

Unlike the Center, GBF forecasts a $1.5 million residual value. Its estimate is based on the following facts: (1) There is no technology on the horizon that would make the Gamma Knife obsolete; (2) the equipment has a physical life estimated to be two-and-a-half times longer than the four-year lease term; and (3) GBF is more skilled in selling used equipment, especially Gamma Knives, than is the Center. GBF's federal-plus-state tax rate is 40 percent, and, if the lease is not written, GBF could invest the funds in a four-year term loan of similar risk yielding 8.0 percent before taxes.

Randall Williams, the Center's chief financial officer, has the final say on all of the business's lease-versus-purchase decisions, but the actual analysis of the relevant data will be conducted by the Center's capital funds manager, Vanessa Seagle. In the past, Randall and Vanessa have more or less agreed on analytical methodologies, but in discussing this lease analysis, they ended up in a heated discussion about the appropriate discount rate to use in the analysis.

Randall argued that the cash flows associated with performing stereotactic radiosurgery are very uncertain. He is convinced that payers are not going to be nearly as generous in the future as they have been in the past in reimbursing for such procedures, so the revenue stream is highly speculative. Accordingly, he thinks that a high discount rate should be used in the analysis. Vanessa, on the other hand, believes that leasing is a substitute for other "financing," which means a blend of debt and equity capital. Consequently, she asserts that the lease-analysis cash flows should be discounted at the Center's corporate cost of capital, 10 percent. However, it is possible that both Randall and Vanessa are wrong.

Both Randall and Vanessa believe that lessees should not blindly accept the first offer made by potential lessors but should conduct a complete analysis from the viewpoint of both parties and then, using this knowledge, negotiate the best deal possible. Thus, knowing the range of lease payments that is acceptable to both parties is important.

There is a possibility that the Center will move to its new radiation facility earlier than anticipated and hence prior to the expiration of the lease. Furthermore, if the neurosurgeon that is the primary user of this equipment leaves the staff and is not immediately replaced, the equipment would be useless. Thus, Randall is considering asking GBF to include a cancellation clause in the lease contract. Under such a clause, the Center would be able to return the equipment to GBF at any time during the lease term after giving a minimum 30-day notice. Before negotiations begin, the Center must assess the impact of such a clause on the riskiness of the lease to both parties and any consequences it might have on the terms of the lease.

In addition to a cancellation clause, Randall is aware that many lessors are now writing per procedure leases, in which the lease payment is tied to the number of procedures performed rather than a fixed amount. Randall wonders what the consequences would be for both the lessee and the lessor if this type of lease were used instead of a conventional lease. GBF has quoted a per procedure lease rate of $7,000 on the basis of an expected annual volume of 100 procedures. However, past experience indicated that volume could easily be as low as 70 or as high as 130 procedures. Considering current charges and reimbursement rates, the Center expects to realize net revenue per procedure of roughly $10,000.

There also has been some discussion about obtaining tax-exempt financing for the Gamma Knife should it be purchased. If so, the cost of tax-exempt (municipal) debt would be only 5 percent. To complicate matters even more, the Center currently has more than $5 million in excess funds invested in marketable securities earning 3 percent, and these funds, rather than debt financing, could be used to purchase the equipment.

Finally, Randall's brother-in-law, who works at GBF, found out that GBF would probably obtain a $1.5 million simple-interest loan that it would use to leverage the lease. The terms of this loan have not been finalized, but the bank has indicated that the interest rate would be in the range of 7 to 9 percent. Such leveraging could affect the Center's ability to negotiate lower lease payments, so it is important to understand the impact of leveraging from the perspectives of both the lessee and the lessor.

Assume that you have been hired as a consultant to recommend a course of action for the Gamma Knife acquisition. Prepare a report that addresses all of the issues raised by the parties involved and makes a final recommendation regarding the acquisition.

SOUTHEASTERN HOMECARE

COST OF CAPITAL

18

SOUTHEASTERN HOMECARE WAS founded in 1992 in Miami, Florida, as a taxable partnership by Maria Gonzalez, MD; Ramon Garcia, RN; and Ron Sparks, LPT. Its purpose was to provide an "at-home" alternative to hospitals and ambulatory care facilities for basic healthcare services provided by physicians, registered nurses, licensed practical nurses, and physical therapists. (For more information on home health services, see the website of the National Association for Home Care & Hospice at www.nahc.org.)

The partnership enjoyed enormous success from the very first day of operations. Even its founders were surprised at how easy it was to establish and run the business. The founding coincided with the search by third-party payers for alternative, and potentially less costly, delivery settings. On the basis of its success in metropolitan Miami, the partnership expanded services into Fort Lauderdale and West Palm Beach and then moved into other metropolitan areas in Florida and across the US Southeast. The partners also expanded their services at each location to include occupational, speech, and rehabilitation therapies.

The founders had sufficient personal resources to start the company, and they had enough confidence in their business plan to commit most of their own funds to the new venture. However, after only six years, the external capital requirements brought on by rapid growth exhausted their personal funds, and they were forced to borrow heavily. Soon, although they still needed external capital to finance growth, the partnership's ability to borrow at reasonable rates was exhausted. Thus, in 2002, they incorporated the partnership, and in 2005, they sold

117

common stock to the public through an initial public offering (IPO). The founders still retain a large, but minority, ownership position in the company, and currently the stock trades in the over-the-counter market.

Southeastern is widely recognized as one of the regional leaders in its industry, and it won an award in 2008 for being one of the 100 best-managed small companies in the United States. The company has two operating divisions: the Healthcare Services Division and the Information Systems Division. The Healthcare Services Division operates Southeastern's home health care services at the company's 22 locations. Because sales and earnings in this division are relatively predictable, the business risk of this division is about average.

The Information Systems Division sells the computer software system that Southeastern designed to control its own operations to other home health care companies. This system combines inventory control, visit scheduling, clinical record keeping, billing and collections, and payroll into a single integrated package. Although the system is excellent, this division competes head-to-head with several major software firms as well as with information services and management consulting firms. Because of this competition, and the rapid technological changes inherent in the information services field, Southeastern's management considers the Information Systems Division to carry more business risk than does the Healthcare Services Division.

Although the company's growth has been exceptional, it has been more random than planned. The founders would simply decide on a location for a new office, run an advertisement in a local newspaper for clinical professionals and clerical employees, send in an experienced manager from one of the established offices, and begin to make money almost immediately. Formal decision structures were almost nonexistent, but the company's head start and its bright, energetic founders easily overcame any deficiencies in its managerial decision-making processes.

However, recent changes in the market for home health care services portend a much more difficult environment in the future. First, relatively generous payment amounts in the 1990s and most of the 2000s produced intense competition in the home health care industry. Other investor-owned home health care firms sprung up like weeds, especially in major cities, and several hospitals in Southeastern's service area, including not-for-profits, began to offer home health care services. Second, the rapid increase in expenditures on home health care services prompted payers to drastically reduce reimbursement amounts just as new capacity came on line. In particular, the Centers for Medicare & Medicaid Services (CMS) has reduced payment rates made under the home health prospective payment system for several years in a row.

Because of these changes, Southeastern's board of directors concluded that the company must start to apply state-of-the-art techniques in both its operations and its corporate managerial processes. As a first step, the board directed the financial vice president (VP) to develop an estimate for the company's cost of capital. The financial VP, in turn, directed Southeastern's treasurer, Clark Ruffin, to prepare and submit a cost-of-capital estimate in two weeks. Clark has an accounting background, and his primary task since taking over as treasurer has been cash and short-term liability management. Thus, he is somewhat apprehensive about his new assignment, an apprehension that is heightened by the fact that one of the board members is a well-regarded University of Florida finance professor.

Clark began by reviewing Southeastern's 2013 financial statements, which are presented in Exhibit 18.1 in simplified form, and by obtaining some selected market data, which are presented in Exhibit 18.2. Next, he assembled the following data for Southeastern.

Long-term-debt:
- Southeastern's long-term debt consists of 7.5 percent coupon, BBB-rated, semiannual payment bonds with 15 years remaining to maturity. The bonds recently traded at a price of $956.31 per $1,000 par value bond. The bonds are callable in five years at par value plus a call premium of one year's interest, for a total of $1,075.
- The founders have an aversion to short-term debt, so the company uses such debt only to fund cyclical working capital needs. The company's financial plan calls for the issue of 30-year bonds to meet long-term debt needs.

Equity:
- Southeastern's last dividend (D0) was $0.17, and its common stock now sells at a price of $5.25 per share. The company has 10 million common shares outstanding.

- Over the last few years, Southeastern has averaged a 20 percent return on equity and has paid out about 50 percent of its net income as dividends.
- Southeastern's historical beta, as measured by several analysts who follow the stock, falls in the range of 1.3 to 1.5.

Capital structure:
- Southeastern's federal-plus-state tax rate is 40 percent.
- Southeastern's target capital structure includes weights of 35 percent long-term debt and 65 percent common stock.

Operating divisions:
- About 60 percent of Southeastern's operating assets are used by the Healthcare Services Division, and 40 percent by the Information Systems Division. Management's best estimate of the beta of its Healthcare Services Division is 1.0.
- Southeastern's divisions are considering the following investment opportunities for next year:

Healthcare Services Division:	*Estimated internal rate of return*
A new office in Naples	9.3%
A new office in Sarasota	9.8%
Information Systems Division:	*Estimated internal rate of return*
A new healthcare record system	12.2%
Expanded billing software	13.2%

Assume that Clark has hired you as a consultant to develop Southeastern's overall corporate cost of capital. You will have to meet with the financial VP—and possibly with the president and the full board of directors (including the founders and the finance professor)—to present your findings and answer any questions.

In addition to the standard analysis, several concerns related to the cost of capital estimate were raised at the last board meeting. First, the board chair noted that the corporate cost of capital estimate is influenced by several factors, some of which are external to the business. She is particularly interested in the impact on the estimated corporate cost of capital of factors that cannot be influenced by managerial actions.

Second, the divisional presidents expressed concern that a single cost of capital will be applied across the company, regardless of any divisional risk differences. Clark has asked you to be sure to address their concerns by developing divisional costs of capital.

Third, the founders of Southeastern are very concerned about the threat posed by home health care businesses started by not-for-profit hospitals because those organizations have both cost (in the sense that they do not pay dividends) and tax advantages. To help assess the threat, Clark has asked you to estimate the cost of capital for an average not-for-profit hospital's home health care business, starting with the information in Exhibit 18.3.

Finally, one of Southeastern's directors has expressed concern over the difference between the company's target capital structure and the current structure as reported on the balance sheet. Clark wondered if this should be a matter for consideration.

Balance Sheet:

Cash and marketable securities	$ 2.5	Accounts payable	$ 1.1
Accounts receivable	5.9	Accruals	1.0
Inventory	1.3	Notes payable	0.2
Current assets	$ 9.7	Current liabilities	$ 2.3
Net fixed assets	32.9	Long-term debt	20.0
		Common stock	20.3
Total assets	$42.6	Total liabilities	$42.6

Income Statement:

Net revenues	$80.6
Cash expenses	71.8
Depreciation	2.8
Taxable income	$ 6.0
Taxes	2.4
Net income	$ 3.6
Dividends	1.8
Additions to retained earnings	$ 1.8

EXHIBIT 18.1
Southeastern Homecare:
2013 Financial Statement
Extracts
(millions of dollars)

**EXHIBIT 18.2
Selected Market Data**

Expected Rate of Return on the Market:
Expected rate of return on the S&P 500 Index = 11.0%

Required Rate of Return on Long-Term Debt of an Average Company:
Yield to maturity on A-rated long-term debt for a company with a beta of 1.0 = 7.0%

Current yield curve on US Treasury Securities:

Term to Maturity	Yield
3 months	2.5%
6 months	3.0
9 months	3.3
1 year	3.5
5 years	4.0
10 years	4.5
15 years	4.8
20 years	5.0
25 years	5.1
30 years	5.2

**EXHIBIT 18.3
Selected Not-for-Profit
Hospital Data**

Average Long-Term Capital Structure:
30 percent debt
70 percent equity (net assets)

Average Cost of Debt:
Interest rate on A-rated tax-exempt bonds = 5.0%

RN TEMPS, INC.

CAPITAL STRUCTURE
ANALYSIS

19

RN TEMPS, INC., franchises "rent-a-nurse" businesses to independent operators throughout the United States. The concept of the business is the same as that of other temporary help services, such as Manpower and Kelly Temporary Services, except that RN Temps deals only with registered nurses. (For an example of a company similar to RN Temps, Inc., see http://interimhealthcare.com.)

The rationale for developing RN Temps is as follows:

1. Many healthcare providers, especially hospitals, have difficulty hiring and retaining nurses, so there is almost always a demand for nursing professionals. Traditionally, hospitals have been the dominant employer of nurses, employing almost 60 percent of the roughly 2.5 million working nurses in the United States. But now nurses have opportunities that were not even dreamed of a generation ago. Registered nurses can work in the nurse practitioner, nurse anesthetist, or critical care or neonatal specialist professions, all of which are in high demand today. In addition, they can work in home health agencies; nursing homes; utilization review departments; physicians' offices or outpatient surgery centers; and a multitude of other nonhospital settings, such as schools. Of all the work settings, hospitals are generally considered to be the least desirable

because of the hard work, rigid work conditions, and irregular working hours. (For more information about the nursing profession, see the American Nurses Association website at www.nursingworld.org.)

2. Providers generally want to minimize fixed costs, so any staffing requirements that may not be permanent in nature are often filled by temporary workers. Also, when vacancies occur among permanent workers, providers often need temporary nurses to carry the load until the vacancies are filled with permanent personnel.

3. Although nursing salaries have increased over the past ten years, real wages have barely kept up with inflation. Furthermore, a large number of nurses have quit the profession for a variety of reasons, including family responsibilities. Many of these nurses are willing to work occasionally but not on a permanent basis. About one in five nurses works part time.

4. Typically, the nurses who want to work on a selective basis have spouses who provide family coverage health insurance. Also, these nurses do not require extensive fringe benefits, such as pension plans or paid vacations, and because they are part-time workers, they are not eligible for unemployment insurance or workers' compensation. Thus, if the average fringe-benefit package paid for permanent nurses is, say, 25 percent of salary, a temporary services company could offer a salary to its nurses 5 percent higher than can providers; could "rent" the nurses out at 5 percent less than it costs providers to hire permanent nurses, including all fringe benefits; and could pocket what remains of the 15 percent spread after administrative costs are paid. Note, however, that the actual rates charged by RN Temps franchisees are related more to local supply-and-demand conditions than to costs.

Franchisees buy the exclusive right to use the RN Temps name within a specified territory from RN Temps, Inc., the franchisor. In addition, franchisees receive marketing and management support from RN Temps as well as the right to lease computers and other office equipment under relatively favorable terms. Finally, franchisees can purchase expendable office supplies directly from RN Temps at substantial savings from retail prices.

To start operations, a franchisee recruits a pool of nurses from the local labor market. Then, when a client needs a temporary nurse, the local manager matches the client's specific needs with a qualified nurse from the pool. The bill for services is sent to the client by the franchisee based on the number of hours—verified by a timecard—that the nurse works for the client. The client has no responsibility for the nurse's salary or fringe benefits; this is all handled by the RN Temps franchisee.

Tiffany Radcliff, a registered nurse from Albuquerque who left the profession to get an MBA from the University of New Mexico, founded RN Temps in 1990. The firm grew rapidly from its base in Albuquerque, first by expanding operations into different cities across the Southwest and then by franchising into other parts of the country. Tiffany was a devout believer in the virtues of equity financing. Although the firm had issued debt periodically, especially to finance company-owned business expansion, Tiffany always used the firm's free cash flow to retire the debt as soon as possible. Recent growth has involved franchising, in which the franchisee puts up the required capital, and hence there has been no need for outside capital for several years.

Tiffany believes that her firm's high-growth days are over. First, numerous companies that offer competing services have appeared on the scene. Second, the number of hospitals, which are her primary clients, has declined over the years since she founded the firm, and a meaningful increase in hospital beds is unlikely in the foreseeable future. Third, many hospitals have created "flexible staffing pools" for nurses, which, for all practical purposes, are in-house temporary work agencies. Finally, many large employers of nurses are recruiting internationally, which lessens the demand for temporary domestic workers. Thus, Tiffany expects the firm's earnings to grow relatively slowly in the future.

Tiffany's financial manager, Paul Duncan, has been preaching for years that RN Temps should use some debt in its capital structure. "After all," says Paul, "everybody else uses debt, and some of our competitors use more than 50 percent debt financing. Also, an underleveraged company is exposed to a hostile takeover because raiders can use the firm's excess debt capacity to finance the bid."

If the firm were to recapitalize, the borrowed funds would be used to repurchase stock in the open market, as the funds are not needed to grow the business. Tiffany's reaction to Paul's prodding is cautious, but she is willing to give Paul the chance to prove his point. Paul has worked with Tiffany for the past six years and knows that the only way he can convince her that the firm should use debt financing is to conduct a comprehensive capital structure analysis.

On the basis of previous conversations, Paul knows that Tiffany has four major concerns about debt financing: (1) the impact on the firm's return on equity (ROE) as reported in the firm's financial statements, (2) the impact on the firm's stock price and corporate cost of capital (CCC), (3) the financial effects of potential changes in business risk of RN Temps, and (4) whether industry averages have any implications for the level of debt financing of RN Temps.

Impact of Financial Leverage on ROE

RN Temps has 10 million shares of common stock outstanding, which are traded in the over-the-counter market. The current share price is $1.20, so the total market value of the firm's equity is $12 million. The book value of equity is also $12 million, so the stock now sells at its book value. The firm's federal-plus-state tax rate is 40 percent. Tiffany owns 20 percent of the outstanding stock, and others in the management group own an additional 10 percent.

Although RN Temps' earnings before interest and taxes (EBIT) is expected to be $3 million in 2014, there is some uncertainty in the estimate, as indicated by the following probability distribution:

Probability	EBIT
0.25	$2,500,000
0.50	3,000,000
0.25	3,500,000

To address Tiffany's first concern, Paul plans to construct partial income statements (beginning with EBIT) for four levels of debt as measured by the book value Total debt/Total assets ratio: zero, 25 percent, 50 percent, and 75 percent. For this analysis, which will not be used to make the actual capital structure decision, Paul intends to use a cost of debt of 10 percent regardless of the amount of debt financing used. Furthermore, any risk implications to stockholders must be identified.

Impact of Financial Leverage on Stock Price and CCC

To address Tiffany's second concern, Paul used a technique to value zero-growth firms at different debt levels. Clearly, the results of this analysis do not apply exactly to RN Temps, which is expected to experience slow growth, as opposed to zero growth, over the coming years. Here are the equations used in the analysis:

$$E = \{EBIT - [R(R_d) \times D]\}(1 - T)/R(R_e)$$
$$V = E + D$$
$$P = (V - D_0)/n_0$$
$$n_1 = n_0 - D/P$$

where

E	=	market value of equity
EBIT	=	earnings before interest and taxes
$R(R_d)$	=	cost of debt
D	=	market (and book) value of new debt
D_0	=	market value of old debt
T	=	tax rate
$R(R_e)$	=	cost of equity
V	=	total market value
P	=	stock price after recapitalization
n_0	=	number of shares before recapitalization
n_1	=	number of shares after recapitalization

Paul arranged for a meeting with an investment banker who specializes in corporate financing for service companies. After several hours, the pair agreed on the estimates for the relationships between the use of debt financing and RN Temps' capital costs, which are shown in Exhibit 19.1. Additionally, Paul obtained industry capitalization data for companies that franchise professional services along with the matching debt ratings on the basis of rough guidance given by Standard & Poor's Ratings Services. These data are provided in Exhibit 19.2.

Business Risk and Industry Averages

Tiffany's third concern is potential changes in the healthcare industry and how they might affect the basic business risk of RN Temps should they occur. To address this concern, Paul produced Exhibit 19.3, which contains leverage/cost estimates at alternative business risk levels. Note that the values in Exhibit 19.3 are for "what if" analysis purposes only. The best current estimates of the financing costs at alternative debt levels are given in Exhibit 19.1.

Tiffany's final concern is whether industry averages have any implications for the level of debt financing of RN Temps. Paul uncovered the following additional industry data: (1) The average healthcare franchise business has a times interest earned (TIE) ratio of 4.0, and (2) RN Temps has cash and marketable securities of $500,000. The average healthcare franchise business has cash and marketable securities on hand equal to 70 percent of its annual interest payment.

Paul also knows that Tiffany is familiar with capital structure theory and will want to know the value of the firm according to the Modigliani-Miller with corporate taxes model and the Miller model. To ease comparisons, Paul assumes that the value of RN Temps, with zero debt financing, is $12 million in both models. He also assumes that the personal tax rates are 15 percent on stock income and 30 percent on debt income.

Put yourself in Paul's shoes and see if you can convince Tiffany that the business should use debt financing.

EXHIBIT 19.1
RN Temps, Inc.:
Estimated Cost of Debt
and Equity at Different
Amounts of Debt
Financing

Amount Borrowed	Cost of Debt	Cost of Equity
$ 0	—	15.0%
2,500,000	10.0%	15.5
5,000,000	11.0	16.5
7,500,000	13.0	18.0
10,000,000	16.0	20.0
12,500,000	20.0	25.0

EXHIBIT 19.2
Healthcare Franchise
Industry Data: Debt
Ratings at Different
Levels of Debt Ratio
(Total debt/Total assets)

Percentile	Debt Ratio	Debt Rating
10th	10%	AAA
25th	25	AA
40th	35	A
Median	50	BBB
60th	65	BB
75th	75	B
90th	82	C

Significant Increase in Business Risk:

Amount Borrowed	Cost of Debt	Cost of Equity
$ 0	—	16.0%
2,500,000	11.0%	17.0
5,000,000	13.0	19.0
7,500,000	16.0	22.0
10,000,000	20.0	26.0
12,500,000	25.0	31.0

Significant Decrease in Business Risk:

Amount Borrowed	Cost of Debt	Cost of Equity
$ 0	—	14.0%
2,500,000	9.0%	14.3
5,000,000	9.5	15.0
7,500,000	10.5	16.0
10,000,000	12.5	17.5
12,500,000	15.5	20.0

EXHIBIT 19.3
RN Temps, Inc.: Estimated Cost of Debt and Equity at Different Amounts of Debt Financing Under Different Business Risk Levels

Capital
Investment

CORAL BAY HOSPITAL

TRADITIONAL
PROJECT ANALYSIS

20

CORAL BAY HOSPITAL is a 250-bed, investor-owned hospital located in Islamorada, Florida, which is known as the "The Sport Fishing Capital of the World." The hospital was founded in 1946 by Rob Winslow, a prominent Florida physician, on his return from service in World War II. Winslow relinquished control of the hospital in 1967 while it was still small and in a relatively quiet setting. However, in recent years, the Florida Keys have experienced a population explosion, which has fostered high economic growth as well as a continuing need for more healthcare services. Today, under a succession of excellent CEOs, the hospital is acknowledged to be one of the leading healthcare providers in the area.

The hospital's management is currently evaluating a proposed ambulatory (outpatient) surgery center. (For more information on ambulatory surgery, see the Ambulatory Surgery Center Association website at www.ascassociation.org.) More than 80 percent of all outpatient surgery is performed by specialists in gastroenterology, gynecology, ophthalmology, otolaryngology, orthopedics, plastic surgery, and urology. Ambulatory surgery requires an average of about one-and-a-half hours to complete: minor procedures take about one hour or less, and major procedures typically take two or more hours. About 60 percent of the procedures are performed under general anesthesia, 30 percent under local anesthesia, and 10 percent under regional or spinal anesthesia. In general, operating rooms are built in pairs so that a patient can be prepped in one room while the surgeon is completing a procedure in the other room.

133

The outpatient surgery market has experienced significant growth since the first ambulatory surgery center opened in 1970. By 1990, about 2.5 million procedures were being performed at stand-alone outpatient centers, and by 2009, the number had grown to more than 20 million. This growth has been fueled primarily by three factors. First, rapid advancements in technology have enabled many procedures that were historically performed in inpatient surgical suites to be offered at outpatient settings. This shift was caused mainly by advances in laser, laparoscopic, endoscopic, and arthroscopic technologies. Second, Medicare has been aggressive in approving new minimally invasive surgery techniques, so the number of Medicare patients utilizing outpatient surgery services has grown substantially. Third, patients prefer outpatient surgeries because they are more convenient, and third-party payers prefer them because they are less costly.

Because of these factors, the number of inpatient surgeries has remained more or less flat over the past 20 years, while the number of outpatient procedures has continuously grown more than 10 percent annually. Rapid growth in the number of outpatient surgeries has been accompanied by a corresponding growth in the number of outpatient facilities nationwide. The number currently stands at about 5,000, so competition in many areas has become intense. Somewhat surprisingly, there is no outpatient surgery center in the hospital's immediate service area, although there have been rumors that local surgeons are exploring the feasibility of a physician-owned facility.

Coral Bay Hospital currently owns a parcel of land adjacent to its facility that is a perfect location for the surgery center. The Hospital bought the land five years ago for $150,000 and last year spent (and expensed for tax purposes) $25,000 to clear the land and put in sewer and utility lines. If sold in today's market, the land would bring in $200,000, net of all fees, commissions, and taxes. Land prices have been extremely volatile, so the hospital's standard procedure is to assume a salvage value equal to the current value of the land. Of course, land is not depreciated for either book or tax purposes.

The surgery center building, which would house four operating suites, would cost $5 million, and the equipment would cost an additional $5 million, for a total of $10 million. For ease, assume that both the building and the equipment fall into the MACRS (modified accelerated cost recovery system) five-year class for tax-depreciation purposes. (In reality, the building would have to be depreciated over a much longer period than the equipment.) The project will probably have a long life, but the hospital typically assumes a five-year life in its capital budgeting analyses and then approximates the value of the cash flows beyond Year 5 by including a terminal, or salvage, value in the analysis. To estimate the salvage value, the hospital typically uses the market value of the building and equipment after five years, which for this project is estimated to be $5 million before taxes, excluding the land value. (Note that taxes must be paid on the difference between an asset's salvage value and its tax book value at termination. For example, if an asset that cost $10,000 has been depreciated down to $5,000 and then sold for $7,000, the firm owes taxes on the $2,000 excess in salvage value over tax book value.)

The expected volume at the surgery center is 20 procedures a day. The average charge per procedure is expected to be $1,500, but charity care, bad debts, managed care plan discounts, and other allowances lower the net patient revenue amount to $1,000. The center would be open five days a week, 50 weeks a year, for a total of 250 days a year. As detailed in Exhibit 20.1, labor costs to run the surgery center are estimated at $918,000 per year, including fringe benefits. Utilities, including hazardous waste disposal, would add another $50,000 in annual costs.

If the surgery center were built, the hospital's cash overhead costs would increase by $36,000 annually, primarily for housekeeping and buildings and grounds maintenance. In addition, the center would be allocated $25,000 of the hospital's current $2.8 million in administrative overhead costs. On average, each procedure would require $200 in expendable medical supplies, including anesthetics. Although the hospital's inventories and receivables would rise slightly if the center is constructed, its accruals and payables would also increase. The overall change in net working capital is expected to be small and hence not material to the analysis. The hospital's marginal federal-plus-state tax rate is 40 percent.

One of the most difficult factors to deal with in project analysis is inflation. Both input costs and charges in the healthcare industry have been rising at about twice the rate of overall inflation. Furthermore, inflationary pressures have been highly variable. Because of the difficulties involved in forecasting inflation rates, the hospital begins each analysis by assuming that both revenues and costs, except for depreciation, will increase at a constant rate. Under current conditions, this rate is assumed to be 3 percent.

When the project was mentioned briefly at the last meeting of the hospital's board of directors, several questions were raised. In particular, one director wanted to make sure that a complete risk analysis, including sensitivity and scenario analyses, was performed prior to the presentation of the proposal to the board. Recently, the board was forced to close a day care center that appeared to be profitable when analyzed two years ago but turned out to be a big money loser. The board does not want a repeat of that occurrence. One of the directors stated that she thought the hospital was putting too much faith in the numbers. "After all," she pointed out, "that is what got us into trouble on the day care center. We need to start worrying more about how projects fit into our strategic vision and how they affect the services we currently offer."

Another director, who also is the hospital's chief of medicine, expressed concern over the impact of the ambulatory surgery center on the current volume of inpatient surgeries. This concern prompted an analysis by the surgery department head, who reported that an outpatient surgery center could siphon off up to $1 million in cash revenues annually. When pressed, the department head estimated that such a reduction in volume could also lead to a $500,000 reduction in annual cash expenses.

To develop the data needed for the risk analysis, Jules Bergman, the hospital's director of capital budgeting, met with department heads of surgery, marketing, and facilities. After several sessions, they concluded that three input variables are highly uncertain: number of procedures per day, average revenue per procedure, and building/equipment salvage value. If another entity enters the local ambulatory surgery market, the number of procedures could be as low as ten per day. Conversely, if acceptance is strong and no competing centers are built, the number of procedures could be as high as 25 per day, compared to the most likely value of 20 per day.

The expected average net patient revenue of $1,000 is a function of the types of procedures performed and the amount of managed care penetration. If surgery severity were high (i.e., if a higher number of complicated procedures than anticipated were performed) and managed care penetration remained low, then the average revenue could be as high as $1,200. Conversely, if the severity were lower than expected and managed care penetration increases, the average revenue could be as low as $800. Finally, if real estate and medical equipment values stay strong, the building/equipment salvage value could be as high as $6 million, but if the market weakens, the salvage value could be as low as $4 million, compared to an expected value of $5 million.

Jules also discussed the probabilities of the various scenarios with the medical and marketing staffs, but after considerable debate no consensus could be reached. To add to the confusion, one member of the medical staff, who had just returned from a University of Michigan executive program on financial management, questioned why the scenario analysis had to be confined to just three scenarios. "Why not five or seven?" he queried. Additionally, the current cost of capital includes an expected inflation estimate of 2 percent that will be used to make a decision today, but future inflation is uncertain and could affect cash flows in the future. Jules said that a good way to assess the impact of uncertain, future inflation on project profitability is to create a table such as the one shown in Exhibit 20.2.

To help with the risk incorporation phase of the analysis, Jules consulted with Mark Hauser, the hospital's chief financial officer, about both the risk inherent in the hospital's average project and how the hospital typically adjusts for risk. Mark told Jules that based on historical scenario analysis data that use worst, most likely, and best case values, the hospital's average project has a coefficient of variation of net present value in the range of 1.0 to 2.0 and that the hospital typically adds or subtracts 4 percentage points to its 10 percent corporate cost of capital to adjust for differential project risk.

Assume that Coral Bay has hired you as a financial consultant. Your task is to conduct a complete project analysis on the ambulatory surgery center and to present your findings and recommendations to the hospital's board of directors.

Position	Annual Salary	FTEs	Total Salary
Executive director	$60,000	1	$ 60,000
Director of nursing	50,000	1	50,000
Accounting clerk	35,000	1	35,000
Collections clerk	30,000	1	30,000
Scheduling clerk	25,000	1	25,000
Registered nurses	60,000	8	480,000
Nursing assistants	30,000	2	60,000
Transcriptionist	25,000	1	25,000
Total			$765,000
Plus 20 percent fringe-benefit allowance			153,000
Total salaries and benefits			$918,000

FTE: full-time equivalent

		Level of Net Patient Revenue Inflation						
		0%	1%	2%	3%	4%	5%	6%
	0%	NPV	NPV	NPV	NPV	NPV	NPV	NPV
Level of	1%	NPV	NPV	NPV	NPV	NPV	NPV	NPV
Cost	2%	NPV	NPV	NPV	NPV	NPV	NPV	NPV
Inflation	3%	NPV	NPV	NPV	NPV	NPV	NPV	NPV
	4%	NPV	NPV	NPV	NPV	NPV	NPV	NPV
	5%	NPV	NPV	NPV	NPV	NPV	NPV	NPV
	6%	NPV	NPV	NPV	NPV	NPV	NPV	NPV

NPV: net present value

NATIONAL REHABILITATION CENTERS

21

STAGED ENTRY ANALYSIS

NATIONAL REHABILITATION CENTERS (NRC) is one of the nation's leading providers of outpatient rehabilitative medicine. It was founded in 1988 in Phoenix, Arizona, by a group of five individuals who recognized the need for cost-effective alternatives to traditional hospital-based rehabilitative services. This vision has become the hallmark of the company, and NRC continues to provide the highest-quality, most cost-effective care available. (For more information on rehabilitative medicine, see the American Academy of Physical Medicine and Rehabilitation website at www.aapmr.org.)

In its quest to lower the costs of rehabilitative services, NRC uses the latest in noninvasive treatment procedures, which reduces direct costs and results in quicker recoveries. In addition, the company encourages patients to begin aggressive rehabilitation as early as possible, which helps them return to normal functioning more quickly than under conventional treatment protocols. In spite of NRC's relatively short history, its strategy has worked wonders, and it quickly expanded from a local to a regional to a national company. Today, NRC is a multibillion-dollar, publicly traded company with nearly 750 locations in all 50 states, Puerto Rico, the United Kingdom, and Australia.

For several years, NRC's board of directors has been considering expanding its service line to include sports medicine. The American College of Sports Medicine defines this field as the physiological, biomechanical, psychological, and pathological phenomena associated with exercise and sports. (For more information on sports medicine, see the American College of Sports Medicine website at http://acsm.org.)

Because there is a considerable degree of commonality between rehabilitative and sports medicine services, expansion into this rapidly growing area of healthcare seems natural.

NRC's board is examining two proposals related to the expansion. Proposal A involves a single, large investment that would immediately give the company a national presence in sports medicine. In essence, all of the current rehabilitation facilities deemed suitable to offer sports medicine services would be renovated, equipped, and staffed as required to offer sports medicine services. The amount of capital investment at each earmarked location would vary significantly, but the average cost is estimated at about $800,000 per facility. With roughly 500 locations identified as being suitable for the sports medicine service line, the estimated cost of Proposal A is in the vicinity of $400 million. Although the profitability analysis of Proposal A is only preliminary, its internal rate of return is thought to be in the range of 20 to 25 percent.

Proposal B, on the other hand, involves a more deliberate, two-stage approach to the expansion. Stage 1 of Proposal B calls for a trial program in which only one of NRC's nine regions would offer sports medicine services. If the results of Stage 1 meet the company's profit targets, Stage 2, which calls for the expansion of sports medicine services into the remaining eight regions, would be implemented.

Proposal A requires a much larger capital investment than does Stage 1 of Proposal B. However, Proposal B is more costly than Proposal A overall, even when the time value of money is considered, because Proposal A's large up-front investment leads to greater efficiencies in contracting, construction, recruitment, and marketing. In spite of Proposal A's cost advantage, several board members are concerned about the wisdom of Proposal A because it requires NRC to make a very large investment in a service line that is new to the company. Other board members, though, see no difference between rehabilitation and sports medicine services, and one board member even said, "healthcare is healthcare."

The primary task at hand now is to evaluate Proposal B, which includes the trial program and possible expansion into all regions. To date, NRC has spent $7 million to develop a sports medicine concept that matches its approach to rehabilitative medicine. Of the $7 million, $2 million have been expensed for tax purposes, while the remaining $5 million have been capitalized and will be amortized over the five-year operating life of Stage 1. According to a specific Internal Revenue Service ruling requested by NRC, if neither Proposal A nor B is implemented, the $5 million could be immediately expensed.

If it decides to go ahead with Stage 1, NRC would immediately spend $2 million to perform local labor-market studies to ensure that the locations identified for the sports medicine program could be staffed. The next step would be to buy the land needed at locations where totally new facilities are required. In total, land acquisition costs, which are assumed to occur at the end of Year 1, are expected to be $10 million. New construction and renovations at the chosen locations would take place during Years 2 and 3, and equipment would be installed during the last quarter of Year 3. Also, additional personnel would be hired as needed at the end of Year 3. The total amount required for new buildings, renovations to existing buildings, and equipment (plus a relatively small amount for recruitment) is estimated to be $50 million. For planning purposes, half of this amount is assumed to be spent at the end of Year 2 and the other half at the end of Year 3.

Although any new buildings actually would fall into the modified accelerated cost recovery system (MACRS) 39-year tax depreciation class for tax purposes, for simplicity both the buildings and equipment needed are assumed to fall into the MACRS seven-year class. Appropriate depreciation allowances are given in Exhibit 21.1. NRC would begin to depreciate the buildings and equipment during Year 4, the year in which the trial sports medicine program would be initiated. The trial program would be evaluated at the beginning of Year 6. If the results are satisfactory, the program would be expanded to the remaining eight regions. If the program does not meet expectations, it would be terminated at the end of Year 8. If terminated, the land would have an estimated market value of $10 million at that time, while the buildings and equipment would have a market value of $30 million.

NRC's marketing department has projected two demand scenarios for Stage 1. If demand for the sports medicine program is poor, total revenues are forecasted to be $40 million for Year 4, the first year of operations. However, if demand is good, revenues are expected to be $60 million. At this point, the best guess is that there is a 50 percent chance of poor demand and a 50 percent chance of good demand. If demand is good, revenues are expected to increase by 6 percent each year after Year 4. If demand is poor, revenue growth is expected to be only 3 percent.

In terms of operating costs, variable costs are expected to be 30 percent of revenues. Fixed costs (other than depreciation), which are expected to total $25 million in Year 4, are forecasted to increase after the initial year of operations at the anticipated overall rate of inflation, 2 percent.

If the board approves Stage 2, NRC would spend an additional $480 million on land, buildings, and equipment to expand into the other eight regions. This expenditure would be evenly split between Years 6 and 7. As shown in the following table, the net cash inflows forecasted for Stage 2 depend on the demand scenario:

	Net Cash Flow		
End of Year	High Demand	Medium Demand	Low Demand
6	($240,000,000)	($240,000,000)	($240,000,000)
7	(240,000,000)	(240,000,000)	(240,000,000)
8	210,000,000	160,000,000	70,000,000
9	228,000,000	170,000,000	75,000,000
10	241,000,000	175,000,000	75,000,000
11	256,000,000	180,000,000	75,000,000
12	500,000,000	350,000,000	150,000,000

Note that the net cash flows have been "bumped up" in Year 9 to reflect the cash flows from those facilities in the test region. Also, note that the project is expected to last beyond Year 12, and an allowance for the value of these future cash flows is embedded in the Year 12 cash flows.

The estimated probabilities of the Stage 2 demand scenarios are related to the response to the Stage 1 trial program. If acceptance is poor in Stage 1, there is a 10 percent probability that demand will be high during Stage 2, a 40 percent probability that demand will be medium, and a 50 percent probability that demand will be low. However, if acceptance during Stage 1 is good, there is a 50 percent probability that demand will be high during Stage 2, a 40 percent probability that demand will be medium, and a 10 percent probability that demand will be low. Of course, these expectations may change over time as new information becomes available. Furthermore, the actual demand scenario for Stage 2 is not expected to be known until midway through Year 8, after the program has been operational nationally for six months.

NRC's current effective income tax rate is 30 percent, and this rate is projected to remain roughly constant into the future. The firm's corporate cost of capital is 10.0 percent, and NRC adjusts this amount up or down by 3 percentage points to adjust for project risk. NRC defines low-risk projects as those that have a coefficient of variation (CV) of net present value less than 0.8, average-risk projects as those that have

CVs in the range of 0.8 to 1.2, and high-risk projects as those that have CVs of more than 1.2.

One of the most important advantages of staged entry is that new information will become available throughout the investment period. NRC's managers recognize the value of this feature and believe that they will have a better estimate of the Stage 2 probabilities and cash flows prior to making the Year 6 investment. Even if Stage 2 is undertaken, there is some possibility that the project could be abandoned at the end of Year 8 if the low-demand scenario materializes. If the project is terminated at that point, the best estimate for the Year 8 abandonment cash flow is $420 million. The uncertainty of whether or not abandonment would occur lies more in the politics than in the economics of the decision. In the past, NRC's managers have not been inclined to admit mistakes and cut losses, so some doubt lingers about whether the abandonment decision would be made even if it is the financially right thing to do at the time.

Assume that you have been hired as a consultant to analyze the situation regarding the sports medicine program and to make a recommendation to NRC's board of directors regarding the best course of action. In addition to a detailed analysis of Proposal B, you have been asked to subjectively compare the relative merits of the two proposals—A and B.

EXHIBIT 21.1
MACRS Depreciation Rates

	Recovery Year				
MACRS Class	1	2	3	4	5
7-year	14.3%	24.5%	17.5%	12.5%	8.9%

Note: For ease, these allowances were rounded to the nearest one-tenth of 1 percent. In actual applications, the allowances would not be rounded.

NORTHWEST SUBURBAN HEALTH SYSTEM

OUTSOURCING DECISIONS

22

NORTHWEST SUBURBAN HEALTH System (the System) is a large not-for-profit healthcare holding company that operates both not-for-profit and for-profit subsidiaries in Chicago's northwest suburbs. The not-for-profit subsidiaries consist of four acute care hospitals (Des Plaines General, Arlington Heights Memorial, Palatine General, and Barrington Community) and one service company (SUPPORT). SUPPORT provides various services, such as food, laundry, and medical waste disposal, to the four hospitals. The single for-profit subsidiary, PROPERTIES, operates several for-profit businesses, but its primary business line is real estate development, particularly medical office buildings.

The System's CEO, Susan Richards, has been thinking about the company's printing situation for some time. The System has a print shop, which currently operates under SUPPORT, that provides some of the printing required by the hospitals, but it does not have the capabilities to do all the work required. As shown in Exhibit 22.1, the System currently (2013) spends about $830,000 a year on commercial contract printing, some of which could be done in-house if the System expanded its printing capability.

Of the roughly $830,000 in total vendor contracts, about $132,000 represents graphics printing—annual reports, brochures, and other promotional material. Most of the graphics printing (about $119,000) could be moved in-house, but about 10 percent of the work (for example, the four-color annual report) would have to continue to be done by outside vendors.

145

Conversely, only about 50 percent of the almost $700,000 in forms printing, or about $349,080, could be moved in-house. Many of the forms require highly specialized equipment, and printing such forms in-house is not cost-effective for businesses, except for very large ones. The System's print contracts (both graphics and forms) with vendors increased in dollar volume by about 5 percent (2 percent volume increase and 3 percent price increase) from 2012 to 2013, and this trend is expected to continue into the foreseeable future.

In 2013, the in-house print shop handled $42,837 in hospital billings. (To avoid any potential problems with SUPPORT's not-for-profit status, the print shop currently performs work exclusively for the System's four not-for-profit hospitals.) The print shop bills for materials only, but because material costs represent, on average, 30 percent of commercial vendors' total billings, it currently does about $42,837/0.30 = $142,790 in annual work on a commercial billing basis. The equipment in the print shop has a current market value of $650,000, and the print shop generates about $40,000 in annual depreciation expense for tax purposes.

To move 90 percent of the vendor graphics printing and 50 percent of the vendor forms printing in-house, the System would have to invest in additional printing equipment. The capital investment necessary for expansion can vary significantly depending on whether new or used equipment is purchased, on the type of main press selected, and on whether only essential or nice-to-have equipment is purchased. Exhibit 22.2 summarizes the equipment capital investment requirements. Note that the old equipment would be retained if the print shop were expanded. Also, the new equipment would generate tax depreciation of about $25,000 per year, and the required delivery van would cost $2,000 a year to operate (in 2013 dollars).

The print shop is located in leased space adjacent to Des Plaines General, the largest of the four hospitals. The cost of this site is $10 per square foot per year. The print shop occupies 2,000 square feet, and hence current building costs are $20,000 in annual lease payments plus $200 per month in utilities and insurance. Unfortunately, this site cannot be expanded, and hence new space is required if the print shop is to increase its capacity. Suitable space in a good location can be leased at the same rental rate ($10 per square foot per year), but the new print shop would require 3,500 square feet, increasing the annual lease cost by $35,000 − $20,000 = $15,000. (Assume that lease payments occur at the beginning of each year.)

Furthermore, the new space would require $30,000 in initial remodeling costs and an additional $100 per month in utilities and insurance costs (in 2013 dollars). Note that all leases are negotiated for a five-year period, so lease payments are not affected by inflation, which is expected to average about 3 percent per year.

The expanded print shop would require an increase in labor costs of $98,400; these costs are summarized in Exhibit 22.3. Labor costs to run the current print shop amount to $50,000 annually, and all current print shop personnel would be retained if the expansion takes place.

After discussing the print shop situation with the System's chief financial officer, Susan defined three possible print shop alternatives:

1. Close the print shop completely, and use outside vendors for all printing.
2. Expand the print shop as envisioned. Essentially, this means expanding the print shop and performing all feasible work in-house. Under this proposal, the print shop would remain under SUPPORT, the System's not-for-profit service subsidiary. Thus, there would be no tax consequences.
3. Expand the print shop as in Alternative 2. However, all printing activities would be transferred to PROPERTIES, the System's for-profit subsidiary. In this situation, capital expenses, such as depreciation and lease payments, would be tax deductible; however, all profits would be taxable. The primary motivation behind this alternative is to permit the print shop to enter the for-profit commercial printing business.

Regarding Alternative 1, many outsiders to the hospital industry would be surprised at the amount of outsourcing that takes place. The business of running a hospital is extremely complicated, and many facets of its operations can be more efficiently run by outside companies that specialize in specific functions. The three most common functions that are outsourced (by number of hospitals) are laundry, housekeeping, and clinical/diagnostic equipment maintenance. However, the list goes on and on. In fact, a significant number of hospitals are now outsourcing some patient care (clinical) services, the most common being anesthesia, emergency department, dialysis, and imaging services. Some hospitals are outsourcing to such a degree that they have created the position of COO—not chief operating officer but chief outsourcing officer.

The System's corporate cost of capital, which is dominated by hospital operations, is estimated to be 8.0 percent. However, the company also computes divisional costs of capital for each subsidiary. SUPPORT, the not-for-profit service subsidiary, has access to municipal debt that currently costs about 5.5 percent. Its target capital structure consists of 60 percent debt and 40 percent equity (fund) financing. Because SUPPORT has a captive business relationship with the System's four hospitals, it has relatively low business risk and, consequently, a relatively low cost of equity of 13.0 percent.

PROPERTIES, the for-profit subsidiary, cannot issue municipal debt. The bulk of its debt consists of mortgage loans provided by banks and insurance companies. Mortgage debt, which is secured by pledged property, has a relatively low interest rate for taxable debt. Currently, this rate is 7.5 percent. The subsidiary's combined federal-plus-state tax rate is 40 percent. Because PROPERTIES competes with other property development companies, its inherent business risk is high, and hence it has a relatively high cost of equity of 17.0 percent. However, PROPERTIES' ability to use real estate as collateral for its debt financing gives it a relatively high debt capacity—about 75 percent. The System's capital budgeting policy guidelines call for all cash-flow analyses to be restricted to a five-year horizon with zero end-of-project salvage values. The rationale is that estimating cash flows any further into the future is just too difficult.

It is now December 2013, and the print shop analysis is due in one week. Thus, for ease, assume that all capital investment cash flows, as well as lease payments for 2014, occur at the beginning of 2014 (the end of 2013). Then, the five years of operating flows occur from 2014 through 2018. Also, the System's capital budgeting policy is to assume that all costs and prices that are not fixed by contract will increase at a 3.0 percent inflation rate. Thus, any 2013 dollar costs must be increased by 3 percent annually beginning in 2014. Furthermore, any 2013 volume amounts must be increased by 2 percent annually beginning in 2014.

In regard to the feasibility of entering the commercial printing business should the print shop be placed into the PROPERTIES subsidiary, Susan discussed the profitability of commercial printing businesses with Mark Stanton, president of the Land of Lincoln Printers Association, the state trade organization. Mark pointed out that the average printer in the United States has a profit margin of 5.5 percent, while the average in the Chicago metropolitan area is barely 4 percent. Return on assets in the industry is 7.5 percent nationwide and 5.2 percent locally.

Estimates regarding the profits that could be earned on commercial printing sales are far from precise, but the best guess is that in 2014 commercial sales could bring in as much as $80,000 in pretax profits (in 2014 dollars). This amount could increase to $100,000 in 2015 (in 2015 dollars), given more time to advertise and build customer relationships. Although very uncertain, the pretax profits that stem from external business are expected to increase by 5 percent per year after 2015, including both volume growth and price inflation. Note that the pretax profit amounts include all costs related to the external printing business except marketing costs, which are estimated at $6,000 in 2014 and are expected to increase at the 3 percent inflation rate.

Finally, the System's purchasing manager has questioned the company's policy regarding external printing contracts: What is the company's current policy, and might a change in policy have a bearing on the decision at hand? The discount rate to use in the analysis has also been an issue under discussion. Susan believes that the discount rate should reflect the divisional placement of the print shop, but some staffers have disagreed with this view. "After all," said one, "the primary factor in choosing a discount rate is the riskiness of the cash flows being discounted."

Assume that you are the administrative resident at Northwest Suburban Health System and have been given the task of analyzing the print shop situation and recommending a course of action. In assigning the project, your preceptor indicated that a risk analysis was appropriate. When asked for more guidance, his response was this: "You know more about this sort of thing than I do; just do it!"

EXHIBIT 22.1
Northwest Suburban
Health System: Printing
Currently Done by
Outside Vendors

	Fiscal Year	
	2012	*2013*
Graphics Printing		
Mercury	$ 85,002.31	$ 7,727.86
Universal Color Graphics	16,982.44	12,588.00
Windy City Press	9,300.00	24,446.00
Northern Illinois Printing	5,628.50	711.94
Pickett Press	3,526.14	2,337.10
Sir Speedy	1,962.58	8,939.50
Northwest Suburban Printing	85.46	0.00
C & S Printing	1,161.00	0.00
Great Lakes Printing Service	0.00	75,292.83
Total graphics printing	$123,648.43	$132,043.23
90% to be brought in-house	$111,283.59	$118,838.91
Forms Printing		
Continuous	$223,826.43	$239,493.82
Stock tab	77,150.41	82,550.50
Labels	68,032.88	65,965.88
Carbon snap	97,563.27	106,283.44
Envelopes	61,096.52	62,435.89
Lab mount	5,095.35	5,126.33
Flat 1/2 side	42,266.69	40,986.45
Special	39,910.37	46,295.47
Oversize	1,458.19	0.00
Special service	1,190.00	2,743.98
Card stock	21,237.40	23,479.11
NCR flat	21,017.01	22,798.19
Total forms printing	$659,844.52	$698,159.06
50% to be brought in-house	$329,922.26	$349,079.53
Total vendor printing	$783,492.95	$830,202.29
Total to be brought in-house	$441,205.85	$467,918.44

Item	Estimated Cost
Two-color press	$ 65,000
Two-color press (small), Model 9860	26,000
Ten-hole drill press	7,800
Futura F-20 folder system	13,000
Collator-stitcher, 12 bin	28,000
Bookmaker, Michael 1000E	5,300
Camera with processor	14,000
Paper plate, AB Dick 148	11,500
Three-knife trimmer	12,000
Infrared dryer systems (2)	5,000
Delivery van	25,000
Miscellaneous items	5,000
Total capital investment	$217,600

EXHIBIT 22.2
Northwest Suburban Health System: Equipment Capital Investment Requirements

Number	Position	Annual Salary
1	Lead printer	$ 42,000
1	Delivery person	25,000
1	Clerical assistant	15,000
	Projected raw-labor expense	$ 82,000
	Plus: 20 percent fringe benefits	16,400
	Total annual incremental labor costs	$ 98,400

EXHIBIT 22.3
Northwest Suburban Health System: Print Shop's Incremental Labor Costs (2013 dollars)

ST. BENEDICT'S TEACHING HOSPITAL

MERGER ANALYSIS

23

THE PATIENT BASE of Lafayette County, Indiana, is currently served by three hospitals: (1) St. Benedict's Teaching Hospital, a not-for-profit, university-related hospital with 525 beds; (2) Wabash Regional Medical Center, a 250-bed for-profit hospital owned by Hospital Associates of America (HAA), a national chain; and (3) Lafayette General, a 400-bed, not-for-profit, acute care hospital owned by Hoosier Healthcare. St. Benedict's and Lafayette are located less than one mile from one another, while Wabash Regional is about five miles away from St. Benedict's, in a newer and more rapidly developing section of the county.

The service area has a total of 1,175 licensed beds, or about 3.5 beds per 1,000 population, which is higher than the national average of about 2.8 beds per 1,000 and much higher than the roughly 2 beds per 1,000 needed under an aggressive utilization management program. Of course, as a tertiary care facility, St. Benedict's receives patients from throughout the state, but the bulk of its patients still come from the local five-county area.

With an excess of hospital beds in the service area, the status quo may not survive the changing healthcare environment. Indeed, Lafayette General has had some tough years recently, as evidenced by its number of discharges, which have fallen to 11,412 in 2013 from 12,055 in 2012 and 12,824 in 2011. Additionally, HAA has been aggressive in building market share in other areas of Indiana, through both acquisitions and hospital expansions. With these factors in place, some consolidation in the local hospital market will likely take place, and the most likely result is the acquisition of Lafayette General by either St. Benedict's or HAA.

Lafayette General operated as a county hospital for more than 50 years and hence developed a reputation for providing healthcare services to the poor. After many years of operating losses, the county concluded that it could no longer afford to operate the hospital. So, in 1987, the county sold the hospital for $1 to Hoosier Healthcare, a not-for-profit managed care organization and provider, which by 2013 had become the state's largest integrated healthcare company.

Hoosier Healthcare's major business line is managed care. Its numerous plans, including HMOs; PPOs; and POS, Medicare, and Medicaid plans, serve more than 1 million members in 25 Indiana counties, encompassing all of the state's major metropolitan areas. In addition to managed care plans, Hoosier Healthcare owns seven different providers: two acute care hospitals, including Lafayette General; one rehabilitation hospital; one mental health facility; one hospice; one home health care provider; and one retirement community.

Lafayette General is the flagship of Hoosier Healthcare's provider network, and the company has kept the hospital in excellent condition in spite of falling inpatient utilization. In fact, in recent years, Lafayette General built the state-of-the-art HeartCare Center and its modern MaternityCare Center. Furthermore, Lafayette General operates a full-service emergency department and a medical helicopter service.

In response to the current situation, St. Benedict's has formed a special committee to consider the feasibility of making an offer to Hoosier Healthcare to acquire Lafayette General. The committee's primary goals are as follows:

1. To place a dollar value on Lafayette General's equity (fund) capital, assuming that the hospital will be acquired and operated by St. Benedict's
2. To develop a financing plan for the acquisition

In addition, the committee has been asked to consider two other issues related to the potential acquisition:

1. What is the best organizational structure for a combined enterprise? Currently, both Lafayette General and St. Benedict's have separate boards of directors and management staffs. Of course, the senior members of the board of Lafayette General currently are Hoosier Healthcare officers.

2. Should the medical staffs of the two hospitals be
    integrated, and, if so, in what way? The medical staff
    of Lafayette General consists of local physicians,
    including many family practice physicians, while the
    medical staff at St. Benedict's is almost entirely made
    up of specialists, and all are members of the local
    university's College of Medicine with responsibilities
    that go well beyond clinical practice.

A new committee will be formed to finalize recommendations
on the above issues should St. Benedict's management agree to move
forward with the acquisition offer, but some preliminary judgments are
sought at this time. As a starting point in the valuation analysis, the committee has obtained historical income statement and balance sheet data
on both hospitals. Exhibit 23.1 contains the data for Lafayette General,
while Exhibit 23.2 provides the data for St. Benedict's. Both sets of statements are abbreviated but still contain the data considered to be most
relevant to the analysis. In addition, some relevant comparative data
are presented in Exhibit 23.3. Finally, relevant market data are shown
in Exhibit 23.4. (Assume that the data in Exhibits 23.3 and 23.4 reflect
late-2013 conditions.)

One of the toughest tasks that the committee faces is the development of Lafayette General's pro forma (forecasted) cash flow statements,
which form the basis of the discounted cash flow valuation. Several basic
questions must be answered before any numbers can be generated. First,
what synergies, if any, can be realized from the merger, and how long
will it take for such synergies to develop? For example, can duplications
be eliminated? Both hospitals have "mercy flight" helicopters, and both
offer full emergency department services, even though the two hospitals
are only one mile apart. And what is the impact of such operational
changes on revenues and costs and hence on the net cash flows that
Lafayette General's assets can produce? Second, once the consolidation
takes place and all synergies have been realized, what is the long-term
growth prospect for Lafayette General's cash flows? Third, what impact
would the acquisition have on St. Benedict's own cash flows? Any
change in St. Benedict's revenues or costs that results from the acquisition must be included in the analysis. The answers to these questions,
and others, form the basis for the pro forma cash flow statements.

Assume that you are the chair of the special committee formed at
St. Benedict's Teaching Hospital to evaluate the potential acquisition.

You must present your findings and recommendations to the hospital's board of directors. Because the case contains far less information than normally available in a merger analysis, especially when the potential merger is friendly, you will be required to make many difficult assumptions to complete your analysis. Although you do not know much about Lafayette General's local market, you do know the current trends in the healthcare industry. Use this knowledge to help make judgments about the case. The quality of many, if not most, real-world financial analyses depends more on the validity of the underlying assumptions than on the theoretical "correctness" of the analytical techniques.

Note that there is no preferred solution to this case, so your case analysis will be judged as much on the assumptions used in the analysis as on the analysis itself. Finally, remember that numerous risk analysis techniques are available that can be used to give decision makers some feel for the risks involved.

	2009	*2010*	*2011*	*2012*	*2013*
Income Statements:					
Inpatient revenue	$ 42.472	$ 46.014	$ 53.410	$ 58.650	$ 59.513
Outpatient revenue	28.314	30.676	35.606	39.100	39.675
Net patient service revenue	$ 70.786	$ 76.690	$ 89.016	$ 97.750	$ 99.188
Nonoperating revenue	1.922	1.515	1.367	1.725	1.048
Total revenues	$ 72.708	$ 78.205	$ 90.383	$ 99.475	$100.236
Patient services expenses	$ 60.245	$ 73.858	$ 81.525	$ 90.645	$ 89.505
Interest expense	3.045	3.147	3.093	3.002	2.980
Depreciation	3.466	3.689	4.395	4.258	6.031
Total expenses	$ 66.756	$ 80.694	$ 89.013	$ 97.905	$ 98.516
Net income	$ 5.952	($ 2.489)	$ 1.370	$ 1.570	$ 1.720
Balance Sheets:					
Cash and investments	$ 2.388	$ 1.538	$ 0.162	$ 0.185	$ 0.198
Accounts receivable	18.860	20.581	20.821	21.570	16.732
Other current assets	4.539	8.475	4.669	2.585	2.898
Total current assets	$ 25.787	$ 30.594	$ 25.652	$ 24.340	$ 19.828
Gross plant and equipment	$102.596	$116.694	$122.611	$133.499	$146.130
Accumulated depreciation	27.243	30.505	34.900	39.158	45.189
Net plant and equipment	$ 75.353	$ 86.189	$ 87.711	$ 94.341	$100.941
Total assets	$101.140	$116.783	$113.363	$118.681	$120.769
Current liabilities	$ 9.182	$ 13.584	$ 5.771	$ 10.689	$ 11.431
Long-term debt	33.572	47.302	50.325	49.155	48.781
Total liabilities	$ 42.754	$ 60.886	$ 56.096	$ 59.844	$ 60.212
Fund balance	58.386	55.897	57.267	58.837	60.557
Total claims	$101.140	$116.783	$113.363	$118.681	$120.769

EXHIBIT 23.1
Lafayette General:
Historical Financial
Statements
(millions of dollars)

	2009	2010	2011	2012	2013
Income Statements:					
Inpatient revenue	$170.195	$198.137	$221.826	$226.944	$251.935
Outpatient revenue	34.225	39.517	46.828	56.226	65.507
Net patient service revenue	$204.420	$237.654	$268.654	$283.170	$317.442
Nonoperating revenue	5.587	8.899	12.193	22.672	9.979
Total revenues	$210.007	$246.553	$280.847	$305.842	$327.421
Patient services expenses	$178.788	$207.596	$231.673	$254.704	$277.938
Interest expense	9.232	10.468	11.983	10.691	9.997
Depreciation	13.289	16.637	19.621	23.286	26.489
Total expenses	$201.309	$234.701	$263.277	$288.681	$314.424
Net income	$ 8.698	$ 11.852	$ 17.570	$ 17.161	$ 12.997
Balance Sheets:					
Cash and investments	$ 17.918	$ 19.862	$ 24.660	$ 27.726	$ 25.220
Accounts receivable	66.212	72.989	99.867	100.297	97.494
Other current assets	12.315	16.771	20.741	20.542	22.757
Total current assets	$ 96.445	$109.622	$145.268	$148.565	$145.471
Gross plant and equipment	$348.288	$341.064	$335.313	$362.152	$400.546
Accumulated depreciation	75.139	76.575	90.056	109.468	123.567
Net plant and equipment	$273.149	$264.489	$245.257	$252.684	$276.979
Total assets	$369.594	$374.111	$390.525	$401.249	$422.450
Current liabilities	$ 42.437	$ 35.061	$ 39.511	$ 37.733	$ 39.817
Long-term debt	146.997	147.038	141.432	136.773	142.893
Total liabilities	$189.434	$182.099	$180.943	$174.506	$182.710
Fund balance	180.160	192.012	209.582	226.743	239.740
Total claims	$369.594	$374.111	$390.525	$401.249	$422.450

Note: The hospital's current target cash balance is $5 million.

	Lafayette	St. Benedict's
Average age of plant	6.8 years	8.5 years
Licensed beds	400	525
Occupancy rate	52.7%	64.2%
Average length of stay	5.5 days	6.6 days
Number of discharges	11,412	19,748
Medicare percent	57.2%	29.7%
Medicaid percent	10.3%	13.0%
Medicare case mix index	1.51	2.13
Gross price per discharge	$11,688	$20,204
Net price per discharge	$5,850	$12,757
Cost per discharge	$5,703	$12,144

EXHIBIT 23.3
Selected Comparative Data

U.S. Treasury Yield Curve:

Maturity	Interest Rate
6 months	3.0%
1 year	3.5
5 years	3.9
10 years	4.5
20 years	5.0
30 years	5.1

EXHIBIT 23.4
Selected Market and Hospital Data

Market Risk Premium:

Historical risk premium	7.0%
Average current risk premium as forecasted by three investment banking firms	6.0%

Market Betas, Capitalization, and Tax Rates of Two Publicly Traded Hospital Companies:

Company	Beta	Debt/Asset Ratio	Tax Rate
Provident Healthcare	1.1	50%	40%
National Health Company	1.2	65%	43%

EXHIBIT 23.4 (continued) Selected Market and Hospital Data

Ratio of Stock Price to EBITDA per Share:

Provident Healthcare	8.5
National Health Company	7.5

Ratio of Total Equity Market Value to Number of Discharges:

Provident Healthcare	$8,000
National Health Company	$7,000

Proportion of Cash to Current Assets:

Large hospital average	5.0%

Days Cash on Hand:

Large hospital average	22 days
St. Benedict's	31 days

EBITDA: Earnings before interest, taxes, depreciation, and amortization

Note: The data in this exhibit are for use in this case only and do not necessarily reflect current market data.

BEACHSIDE HEALTH PARTNERS

JOINT VENTURE ANALYSIS

24

BEACHSIDE HOSPITAL (the Hospital) is a 320-bed, acute care, not-for-profit hospital located in Myrtle Beach, South Carolina. It is well known as a leader in new technology and hence draws patients from as far away as Georgetown to the south and Wilmington, North Carolina, to the north. The Hospital contracts with the Grand Strand Radiology Group (the Group) to provide radiology services for its patients. Basically, the Hospital furnishes the radiology equipment and technicians and performs the tests, while the physicians in the Group "read" the results. Because the Group bills patients separately for the readings, there is no direct payment from the Hospital to the Group.

Assume it is now 1988. At the end of one of the monthly medical staff meetings, Dr. George Brigham, head of the Group, presented a proposal to Mary Cohen, the Hospital's CEO. The Group wants to form a partnership with the Hospital to purchase a biliary lithotripter, a device that uses shock waves to crush gallstones. Lithotripsy emerged in the early 1980s as a noninvasive way to shatter kidney stones: Patients are placed in a water bath, partially anesthetized, and then subjected to repeated focused blasts of shock waves transmitted through the water. By 1988, renal lithotripsy was well developed, and researchers were beginning to apply the same technology to gallstones, which are extremely common and affect about 20 million Americans. With about 300,000 cholecystectomies (surgical removal of the gallbladder) performed annually, biliary lithotripsy offers the prospect of a painless, noninvasive, and cost-saving alternative to surgery.

The biliary lithotripter, which costs about $1 million, has not yet received approval from the Food and Drug Administration (FDA), and hence it does not qualify for Medicare/Medicaid reimbursement. However, the FDA has granted approval to begin clinical trials. If these trials satisfy the FDA standards for efficacy and safety, biliary lithotripter manufacturers would be permitted to freely market the technology. (For more information on the approval process, see the FDA website at www .fda.gov.) The Group would be involved in lithotripter usage because radiologists must read the ultrasound images that are used to locate the stones and confirm that the treatment has been effective.

Mary had recently read an article on biliary lithotripsy, and she is supportive of the idea. Furthermore, Dr. Brigham mentioned that he had talked to the president of Medical Equipment International (MEI), the developer of the biliary lithotripter. During the conversation, MEI promised to give the Hospital exclusive purchase rights in its service area during the trial period, which is a process expected to take about two years.

The idea of being an exclusive provider of gallstone lithotripsy appeals to Mary, even if it only lasts for two years. First, by offering this procedure, the Hospital is reinforcing its position as the regional leader in new technology. Second, an early start would position the Hospital as the leading provider if the technology became available to competing hospitals. Mary does not believe that the Hospital's board of trustees would be willing to bear the entire risk of the purchase, but she thinks it might be willing to go along with a joint venture. Thus, Mary asked Dr. Brigham to look into the matter further and develop a specific joint venture proposal.

Mary had almost forgotten the matter when, two months later, Dr. Brigham appeared with the following proposal (Exhibit 24.1 contains a summary of the proposed financing):

1. A separate business entity, Beachside Health Partners (the Partnership), would be formed.
2. The Partnership would have two general partners: the Group and the Hospital. The Group would put up $300,000 in capital and retain 60 percent management control, while the Hospital would furnish $200,000 in capital and obtain 40 percent control. (The Group is incorporated, but it files federal income taxes as an S corporation. It would

incorporate a subsidiary S corporation for the sole purpose of investing in the Partnership. S corporations pay no federal income taxes. Rather, as in a partnership, the income is constructively prorated among the owners and taxed as ordinary income.)

3. Twenty-five limited partnerships would be offered to local physicians for $20,000 each. The limited partners (the LPs) would have no liability beyond their $20,000 investments but, on the other hand, would have no control rights. (The Partnership is purposely restricted to 25 limited partners because a larger number would require a more complicated partnership registration procedure with the State of South Carolina.)

4. An additional $1 million would be obtained from South Carolina Bancorp in the form of a five-year term (amortized) loan carrying an interest rate of 8 percent. The bank would require the Partnership to pledge the equipment as collateral for the loan. In the event of default by the Partnership, the market value of the equipment would first be used to offset the principal balance, and then the Group would be liable for 60 percent and the Hospital for 40 percent of any remaining balance.

The $2 million initial capital infusion would be just sufficient to purchase and install the lithotripter and to pay the consulting, legal, and accounting costs associated with forming the Partnership. The Hospital would lease the Partnership the space for the lithotripter, furnish the technical support required to operate the equipment, and handle billing and collections. Of course, all services provided to the Partnership by the Hospital would be handled at arm's length, and hence the Partnership would pay the Hospital prevailing market rates for the services provided.

The Partnership itself would not be taxed, but its distributions represent income and as such would be taxed on the basis of each partner's tax status. The distributions to the Hospital would be nontaxable because the joint venture is consistent with the Hospital's not-for-profit status. The distributions to the Group and to the LPs would be taxed as ordinary income. However, about 50 percent of the distributions would represent a return of capital (depreciation cash flow), which is not taxed, and hence taxable investors would pay taxes at an effective rate of only about 20 percent.

The cash flows from the Partnership would be distributed according to the following plan:

1. The Partnership would distribute all earned net cash flow to the partners at the end of each year.
2. At the end of the first year, the general partners would receive 30 percent of the cash flow and the LPs would receive 70 percent. Following the distribution at the end of each year, the total accumulated dollar return provided to the LPs would be calculated. If this amount is less than the LPs' total investment, they would continue to receive 70 percent of the cash flow in the following year.
3. In the years succeeding the year in which the LPs recover their initial investment, 50 percent of the cash flow would be distributed to the general partners, while 50 percent would go to the LPs.
4. The cash flow allocated to the general partners would be distributed proportionally to the Group and to the Hospital on the basis of each partner's relative investment: 60 percent would go to the Group and 40 percent to the Hospital.

Of course, the key to a sound financial analysis is good cash flow estimates. Mary and Dr. Brigham devoted an entire day to the cash flow estimation process, and many other individuals provided input. If the joint venture gets off the ground, the lithotripter would be in operation by the end of the year (Year 0). The equipment would be available for 50 weeks each year, and the best estimate is that four procedures would be performed per week during the first year (Year 1).

Although biliary lithotripsy has only been approved for trials, several third-party payers have expressed an interest in supporting the testing. If the technology is successful, lithotripsy would significantly lower future costs for the treatment of gallstones. Based on discussions with selected payers, the Partnership is expected to receive $5,000 per procedure on average. Thus, the net revenue in Year 1 is forecasted to be 4(50)($5,000) = $1,000,000. Physician and public awareness would increase after the first year, and hence volume is projected to increase to five procedures per week during Year 2. Although FDA approval would mean additional utilization by Medicare/Medicaid patients in Year 3, at least one competing hospital would likely have its own lithotripter by this time. Thus, volume is expected to fall back to four procedures per week in Year 3, to three procedures per week in Year 4, and to two procedures per week in Year 5.

Projecting the trend for net revenue per procedure is difficult. On the one hand, it might be possible to increase the charge for biliary lithotripsy by the overall inflation rate, or even more. But on the other hand, FDA approval would mean that Medicare/Medicaid patients would join the patient mix, and reimbursement for their care is often set well below chargemaster prices; indeed, such payments could be below costs. Because these factors tend to offset one another, no inflation adjustments will be applied to revenue estimates.

Technology is moving quickly in this area, so assessing whether the lithotripter would have an economic life of more than five years is very difficult. For the same reason, estimating the machine's salvage value at the end of five years is also difficult. Because of the uncertainties involved, Mary and Dr. Brigham agreed to assume a five-year life for the Partnership and a zero salvage value for the equipment.

Exhibit 24.2 contains the forecasted cash flow statements for the Partnership for Years 1 and 2. Note the following points:

1. Technician costs are estimated at $100 per procedure, so total technician support for Year 1 is $(4)(50)\$100 = \$20,000$.
2. Clerical costs are estimated at $50 per procedure, so total clerical expense for Year 1 is $(4)(50)\$50 = \$10,000$.
3. Technician and clerical salaries are expected to increase at an annual rate of 5 percent.
4. Rent, insurance, and marketing expenses are forecasted to be $15,000, $10,000, and $5,000, respectively, in Year 1. These costs are expected to increase at the projected inflation rate of 5 percent.
5. Expendable supplies are estimated to cost $20 per procedure, and hence the Year 1 total supplies cost is $(4)(50)\$20 = \$4,000$. Furthermore, the cost of expendables is expected to increase at the 5 percent inflation rate.

6. The service contract on the lithotripter is expected to cost $50,000 in Years 1 and 2, $75,000 in Years 3 and 4, and $100,000 in Year 5. These costs increase over time because cumulative usage increases the need for maintenance and parts replacement.

7. The Partnership will have to pay property taxes on the equipment, currently estimated to be $23,000 in Year 1, $24,000 in Year 2, $25,000 in Year 3, $26,000 in Year 4, and $27,000 in Year 5.

8. The Partnership's administrative expenses are estimated to be $30,000 per year. These expenses consist of accounting and legal fees as well as reimbursement for management time spent on Partnership business. These costs are expected to increase at the 5 percent inflation rate.

9. Principal and interest expenses are based on annual amortization of an 8 percent, five-year loan of $1,000,000.

10. Miscellaneous expenses, which consist of the costs involved in the semiannual partners meeting, forms printing, expendable clerical supplies, and so on, are expected to be a constant $20,000 over the next five years.

Mary and Dr. Brigham are most concerned about the estimates for weekly volume, and hence they spent a great deal of time developing the following data:

	Weekly Volume				
Case	Year 1	Year 2	Year 3	Year 4	Year 5
Worst	3	4	3	2	1
Most likely	4	5	4	3	2
Best	5	6	5	4	3

These estimates assume that the biliary lithotripter will meet the manufacturer's expectations regarding efficacy and safety. However, any problems in this regard could mean that the trials could be curtailed or even discontinued. Even if the trials were completed, failure to obtain final FDA approval would mean a whole new ball game.

Assuming no problems occur during the trial and subsequent FDA approval, the best estimates for the probabilities of the above scenarios are 25 percent for the best and worst cases and 50 percent for the most likely case.

The current yield on 20-year T-bonds is 5 percent. Furthermore, a local brokerage firm estimated the market risk premium to be 5 percentage points. Thus, according to the Capital Asset Pricing Model (CAPM), the current required rate of return on an average-risk (large publicly traded company with a beta equal to 1.0) stock investment is 10 percent.

In addition to the efficacy concerns, all parties have expressed concern over two other issues. First, are there any indirect costs or benefits (i.e., costs or benefits that do not appear in the estimated cash flows) to any of the parties to the venture? Second, does the Partnership raise any legal or ethical issues for any of the parties?

Assume that you have been hired as a consultant to examine the feasibility of the proposed joint venture. You must assess the situation and prepare a report for the Hospital and the Group. Mary and Dr. Brigham know that the joint venture will never be successful unless all parties are satisfied with the financial arrangements. Thus, they believe that an impartial analysis should be conducted to assess the risk/return potential for each party. Furthermore, if any of the parties do not appear to be treated fairly under the initial proposal, they would seek recommendations that would increase overall fairness and hence give the proposal a better chance of success.

In beginning your analysis, you recognize that there are several different cash flow/discount rate formats available for valuing businesses. In essence, the partnership analysis is merely business valuation—but from the perspective of different classes of equity participants. To allow the analysis to include multiple equity perspectives, it is necessary to structure the cash flows using the free-cash-flow-to-equityholders method. Here, the focus is on the cash flows that are available for distribution to equityholders, so interest expense (and any other debt flows) must be subtracted from the cash flow stream. (Note that this format differs from a typical capital budgeting analysis, in which debt flows are not considered.) Because the estimated net cash flows are equity flows, they must be discounted by a cost of equity. (Typical capital budgeting cash flows are operating cash flows and hence are discounted by the corporate cost of capital, adjusted for individual project risk.)

You also note that sensitivity analysis is not very useful in this situation because the unique cash flow distribution system confounds such an analysis. In addition, internal rate of return, although useful for the base case, breaks down in a scenario analysis because some scenarios create non-normal cash flows. Thus, you plan to use standard scenario analysis techniques for your risk analysis, with net present value as the profitability measure. Furthermore, because the purpose of scenario analysis is to assess risk, rather than incorporate it, you plan to use a constant 10 percent discount rate for all partners in the scenario analysis.

Finally, you can't seem to shake the feeling that something might go wrong during the clinical trials. In fact, a nurse who had worked as a clinical consultant for MEI before moving to Myrtle Beach has expressed some concern about the effectiveness of biliary lithotripsy. "Lithotripsy may work well on kidney stones, but I'll bet you a dollar to a doughnut that it won't work on gallstones," she was reported to say. Thus, you want to ensure that the analysis considers at least one scenario in recognition that the technology might fail to produce the desired results.

EXHIBIT 24.1
Beachside Health Partners: Partnership Financing Summary

Capital Contribution	General Partners	Limited Partners	Debt Financing
$ 300,000	Group		
200,000	Hospital		
500,000		25 @ $20,000 each	
1,000,000			SC Bancorp
$2,000,000			

	Year 1	Year 2
Net revenues	$1,000,000	$1,250,000
Cash operating costs:		
Technician support	$ 20,000	$ 26,250
Clerical support	10,000	13,125
Rent	15,000	15,750
Insurance	10,000	10,500
Marketing expenses	5,000	5,250
Expendable supplies	4,000	5,250
Service contract	50,000	50,000
Property taxes	23,000	24,000
Administrative expense	30,000	31,500
Principal repayment	170,456	184,093
Interest expense	80,000	66,363
Miscellaneous expenses	20,000	20,000
Total expenses	$ 438,456	$ 453,394
Partnership net cash flow	$ 561,544	$ 796,606

EXHIBIT 24.2
Beachside Health Partners: Forecasted Cash Flow Statements

25

BEDFORD CLINICS
PRACTICE VALUATION

United Health Services Corporation

UNITED HEALTH SERVICES Corporation (UHSC) is a large integrated healthcare business that serves Northern and Central California. In response to healthcare reform, UHSC has been acquiring primary care practices to capture market share. The basic competitive strategy has been to select geographically well-placed practices that will attract and retain patients. UHSC believes this strategy will be critical in the shift to population health management.

Initial acquisitions were not entirely successful, primarily because of overvaluation of downstream revenue. In essence, UHSC overpaid for practices in anticipation of higher referrals and revenue after acquisition. Most were small, one-physician practices and UHSC quickly learned that typically they had insufficient patient volume to cover the substantial fixed costs of running a practice, had a payer mix of more than half from less profitable Medicare and Medicaid sources, included a physician who was not seeing an adequate number of patients per day, and paid insufficient attention to the efficient operation of the practice. On the plus side, they typically had a loyal patient base and were usually seen as providing an important service in the community.

Perhaps as a result of the less-than-successful experience with small primary care practices, UHSC next acquired a much larger practice—Anderson Clinic. The large patient volume, the lucrative payer mix, and the busy physicians have made Anderson Clinic a financial success for UHSC. However, there have been substantial problems with this acquisition as well. Most important, changing the culture of a large practice has been difficult. The majority of Anderson Clinic physicians have been with the practice a long time and resisted many of the clinical and customer processes introduced by UHSC. Many implementation problems have occurred, and complaints from a large number of physicians have required a lot of UHSC management time. One UHSC manager said, "Anderson gives us most of our profit, but it also gives us most of our headaches."

This less-than-successful experience with small primary care practices and a large practice prompted UHSC to review its practice acquisition strategy. After several months of study, UHSC decided that, although it can help to reduce practice costs and increase efficiency, the revenue side of the practice is what's most important. Thus, UHSC has established five criteria for evaluating acquisition of a practice:

1. Adequate patient volume for the number of providers
2. Viable payer mix
3. Physician productivity
4. Effective operations, including revenue cycle management, pricing of services, coding and documentation, and service mix
5. Qualitative factors, including patient referrals from customer service, organizational culture, quality improvement, and community relations

These criteria have resulted in UHSC adopting a strategy of acquiring "not-too-big and not-too-small" primary care practices. These multiphysician practices are not as financially lucrative as larger practices such as the Anderson Clinic, but incorporation of the practices into the organization has been much easier. Thus, management has decided that this type of practice is what works best for UHSC and has been looking to acquire more practices of this type.

In the Bedford region of Central California, UHSC has acquired several practices in the southern end but does not yet have a practice in the northern end. UHSC practices provide general primary care services only, but UHSC is exploring provision of some specialty services, such as pain clinics. UHSC plans to try some specialty services in a few practices to determine whether there is a business case to support an extensive rollout.

Bedford Clinics

One of the primary care practices that UHSC wants to acquire is Bedford Clinics, which is located in the northern end of the Bedford region. Several years ago, UHSC had targeted Bedford Clinics for acquisition but attempts to interest the two founding partners had failed. At the time, they had no interest in being purchased by a larger organization.

Nevertheless, Bedford Clinics was too inviting a takeover target to be overlooked for long. UHSC believes that acquisition of the practice would attract and retain new patients to the network; increase referrals to other UHSC services; and better prepare UHSC for the new, post-healthcare reform funding models. Bedford would benefit from access to a larger network and greater net revenue from the UHSC expertise in boosting physician productivity. In addition, some of the UHSC senior managers know the two Bedford Clinics founding partners, having served on various community committees together. "The Bedford docs see things the way we see them," a UHSC senior manager recently said. For these reasons, UHSC has continued to keep an eye on Bedford, following its physicians and business activities.

Today Bedford Clinics operates two walk-in clinics and consists of five physicians—three are board certified in family practice and two in internal medicine. Three work full time and two work half time, resulting in four full-time equivalent (FTE) physicians. Bedford Clinics is organized as a for-profit corporation, but for tax purposes the business is classified as an S corporation. (In an S corporation, the business pays no taxes. Rather, the corporation's taxable income is constructively distributed to the owners, who pay personal taxes on the income.)

Bedford Clinics was founded ten years ago by two physicians (the part timers) who wanted to have more free time than their solo practices allowed. Initially, Bedford Clinics had only one location, but a second was recently added. The downtown clinic, whose patients predominantly come directly from work sites, is open Monday through Friday from 8 a.m. to 2 p.m. The midtown clinic, whose patients mostly come from home, is open Monday through Saturday from 8 a.m. to 8 p.m. The midtown clinic also provides a few specialty services, including a diabetes clinic. Both clinics are open 52 weeks per year. Exhibit 25.1 provides the average number of visits by day for the two clinics, and Exhibit 25.2 shows the current payer mix. With the current medical and clerical staffs, as well as clinic space, Bedford's patient volume can grow as much as 50 percent without the need for additional personnel or facilities.

The five physicians who make up Bedford Clinics own the business. However, the two founding partners control the business: Each has a 35 percent ownership stake. The remaining three partners each own 10 percent of the business. Because the founding partners are looking to fully retire in the near future, they would like to sell the business. The remaining partners are less enthusiastic about selling out, but as minority owners their alternatives are limited.

The most recent income statement of the business is provided in Exhibit 25.3. Note that the statement uses the effective average tax rate applicable if Bedford were to file as a C corporation. A condensed balance sheet is contained in Exhibit 25.4. If UHSC acquires Bedford Clinics, it would maintain the current debt ratio into the foreseeable future and has an agreement with a lending institution to borrow funds at a rate of 6 percent. In addition to assets used in the day-to-day operations of the business, Bedford holds nonoperating assets (marketable securities and investment properties). The marketable securities represent a "rainy day" fund, while the investment properties were acquired to diversify the asset holdings and revenue stream of Bedford.

Bedford Clinic's cost structure, listed in Exhibit 25.4, is expected to hold in the immediate future, with fixed costs (including depreciation) increasing at a 2 percent annual rate. Furthermore, Bedford Clinics will have to invest roughly $25,000 each year (in Year 1 dollars) in new equipment. Inflation is expected to increase these capital investment amounts by 2 percent per year.

Wilde and Sullivan

To ensure that it did not overpay for a primary care practice again, UHSC decided to retain the services of Wilde and Sullivan, a California firm that specializes in physician practice valuation and appraisal. Heidi Wilde, the managing partner, had recently valued four practices in the Central California region that includes Bedford, so she decided to use this experience as a starting point in estimating the value of Bedford Clinics to UHSC. Selected data for these acquisitions are shown in Exhibit 25.5.

First, Heidi estimated the expected revenue growth rate for the short term (Years 1–5) and the long term (Years 6 and beyond). In reviewing the data in Exhibit 25.5, Heidi noted that Bedford Clinics and all of the recent practice acquisitions are located in the same geographic area, so it's reasonable to assume that Bedford Clinics faces the same estimated long-term (Years 6 and beyond) revenue growth rate of 2 percent. However, Heidi has found that the short-term (Years 1–5) revenue growth rate of a particular practice depends on the current level of physician productivity: Clinics with relatively low physician productivity have higher short-term (Years 1–5) revenue growth rates because of room for productivity increases. Heidi also believes that there is opportunity for improved coding and documentation, better revenue cycle management, and an updated chargemaster at Bedford Clinics.

Next, Heidi assembled the information required for use of the discounted cash flow (DCF) approach, including the estimated required rate of return on an equity investment in Bedford Clinics. Little market data about primary care practices are available for guidance, but the current yield on long-term Treasury bonds is 4 percent, while the historical risk premium on the market, which reflects the premium on an average-risk common stock investment, is about 5 percent. Of course, there are significant risk and liquidity differences between direct ownership of a relatively small group practice and ownership of the stock of a large, publicly traded corporation. UHSC also informed Heidi that it estimates its tax rate will be 20 percent for the foreseeable future.

In addition to the DCF approach, Wilde and Sullivan use three market multiple methods to value medical practices: physician FTEs, net patient revenue, and EBITDA (earnings before interest, taxes, depreciation, and amortization). In these methods, a proxy for value is multiplied by a market-determined factor that best expresses the relationship of that proxy to equity value.

With this information at hand, Heidi's task is to estimate the value of Bedford Clinics to UHSC and recommend whether UHSC should make the acquisition.

EXHIBIT 25.1
Bedford Clinics: Current
Average Number of
Visits by Day and Clinic

	Downtown	*Midtown*
Monday	39	57
Tuesday	33	46
Wednesday	33	43
Thursday	34	44
Friday	33	28
Saturday	—	37
Total	172	255

EXHIBIT 25.2
Bedford Clinics:
Current Payer Mix

Medicaid	9%
Medicare	21%
Private insurance	52%
Out-of-pocket	18%
Total	100%

EXHIBIT 25.3
Bedford Clinics:
Current Free
Cash Flow Statement

Net revenues	$1,491,791
Operating expenses:	
Fixed	719,997
Variable	349,079
Total operating expenses	1,069,076
EBIT	$ 422,715
Interest expense	25,575
EBT	$ 397,140
Taxes	119,142
Net profit	$ 277,998

EBIT: earnings before interest and taxes; EBT: earnings before taxes

Notes: 1. Operating expenses include depreciation of $11,070.
2. Capital expenditures for the year were $15,000.

Assets:	
Cash and cash equivalents	$ 73,475
Marketable securities	42,399
Accounts receivable	85,702
Medical and administrative supplies	9,890
Current assets	$ 211,466
Net plant and equipment	1,689,524
Investment properties	450,461
Total assets	$2,351,451
Liabilities and Owner's Equity:	
Notes payable	$ 352,718
Owner's equity	1,998,733
Total liabilities and equity	$2,351,451

Note: Adjustments to the amount of debt in the capital structure occur at year-end. Thus, interest expense on the income statement can be calculated from the previous year's balance of notes payable.

EXHIBIT 25.4
Bedford Clinics: Current Balance Sheet

	Alvarez Family Health	Johnson Walk-In Center	South Side Clinic	Wilson Internal Medicine
Patient visits	5,600	34,000	40,000	170,000
Net patient revenue	$380,000	$2,400,000	$2,700,000	$13,000,000
EBIT	$159,000	$520,000	$600,000	$2,000,000
Depreciation	$20,000	$80,000	$90,000	$800,000
Full-time physicians	1	2	4	20
Part-time physicians	0	6	3	4
Estimated Year 1–5 revenue growth rate	5%	4%	3%	2%
Price	$800,000	$6,000,000	$7,000,000	$44,000,000

EBIT: earnings before interest and taxes

EXHIBIT 25.5
Wilde and Sullivan: Selected Data for Recent Acquisitions of Primary Care Practices in the Bedford Region

SHASTA FACULTY PRACTICE

26

PHYSICIAN EXTENDER ANALYSIS

SHASTA FACULTY PRACTICE (the Practice) is the not-for-profit corporation that controls the clinical operations of the medical faculty of Shasta University. The Practice provides all physician services for Shasta Health System (the System), which consists of six hospitals plus supporting services that, in total, provide the entire continuum of care. The main inpatient facility is a 650-bed tertiary care academic medical center, although the System also owns two rural 50-bed hospitals, one 125-bed community hospital, and a 250-bed long-term care facility. In addition to inpatient facilities, the System owns multiple outpatient clinics and has established joint ventures with several other outpatient providers.

The Practice's vice president for outpatient services, Dr. Rudy Mason, is exploring the use of physician extenders in the clinics as a way of enhancing physician productivity and, ultimately, the Practice's profitability. In recent years, the role of physician extenders has evolved to the point where they are having a considerable impact on the delivery of care in many different settings. For example, physician extenders can perform more than 80 percent of primary care physicians' patient care duties, including taking medical histories; performing physical examinations; diagnosing and treating illnesses; ordering and interpreting laboratory tests; and, in most situations, prescribing medications. Although the term *physician extender* remains widely used, other terminology applied to such individuals includes *advance practice professionals*, *mid-level providers*, and *nonphysician providers* (NPPs).

179

The use of extenders allows physicians to treat more and higher-acuity patients, therefore expediting patient flow and increasing revenues. Also, because compensation for physician extenders is less than that for physicians, costs per patient visit can be lowered. In addition to the obvious productivity and economic benefits, studies indicate that patient satisfaction improves when physician extenders are used. In essence, they are willing (and often able) to spend more time with each patient than physicians usually do. This extra attention typically results in better quality of care (real or perceived) and higher patient satisfaction.

However, as the role of physician extenders expanded, it was inevitable that some conflicts would arise. The increasing recognition by third-party payers that extenders are as acceptable as physicians in providing many services means extenders are a potential source of direct competition for physicians. Still, physicians at many solo and group practices are using extenders to supplement and complement their work. (The Medical Group Management Association reported in 2010 that 92 percent of physician-owned practices use extenders. Furthermore, these practices reported higher median physician compensation.) Adding to the extender-use trend, predicted shortages in primary care physicians (roughly 65,000 by 2025, according to the Association of American Medical Colleges) means that extenders will have to fill the physician void to prevent reduced access to primary care.

The two main types of physician extenders are advanced registered nurse practitioners (NPs) and physician assistants (PAs). Although NPs and PAs often perform similar tasks, their training and certification requirements differ. NPs must be licensed in the state in which they practice. To acquire such licensure, an individual must be licensed as a registered nurse (RN), meet additional education and practicum requirements that historically led to a master's degree, and pass a national certification examination in one of several specialized areas. Now, however, most nursing schools that offer nurse practitioner education are transitioning to programs that lead to doctor of nursing practice (DNP) degrees. This trend has created an expectation that, at some future date, the DNP degree will become a requirement for certification. (For more information on NPs, see the website of the American Association of Nurse Practitioners at www.aanp.org.)

PAs must graduate from an accredited physician assistant educational program and then obtain certification by the National Commission on Certification of Physician Assistants. The educational training for a PA is similar to that of a physician, but much shorter—historically only two years. Although PA programs traditionally offered either associate or bachelor's degrees, most programs today are at the master's level. (For more information on PAs, see the website of the American Academy of Physician Assistants at www.aapa.org.)

Although it may appear on the surface that NPs and PAs are perfect substitutes for one another, the differences in educational background create differences in philosophies of care. Because NPs follow the nursing model of care, which focuses on health education and counseling as well as disease prevention, they typically have a special concern for the overall health and welfare of patients. PAs, on the other hand, generally follow the medical model of care, which focuses on diagnosis and treatment. Of course, these are generalizations that do not necessarily apply to specific individuals. Although most NPs and PAs practice in primary care settings, others specialize in such areas as dermatology, pediatrics, geriatrics, anesthesiology, surgery, and emergency medicine.

The practice status of physician extenders has been, in large part, driven by state law. Historically, some states allowed NPs to practice independently, while others mandated some physician involvement (collaborative or supervisory). With PAs, most states required that a physician be physically present (or electronically available) when a PA treats a patient. In addition, many states allowed NPs to prescribe all medications independent of physician supervision, while the ability of PAs to prescribe medications was much more limited. However, the Balanced Budget Act of 1997 removed many of the limitations imposed by individual states. Now, both NPs and PAs are allowed to practice without the immediate availability of a supervising physician. Note, however, that NPs are allowed to practice under their own licenses, while PAs must practice under the license of a physician.

The reimbursement of physician extenders, like all reimbursement for healthcare services, is complicated by the fact that there are many different third-party payers using different payment methodologies. For purposes of this case, assume that all payers use the same system as Medicare, which recognizes several different situations in which extenders provide services.

In general, Medicare pays extenders in all settings 85 percent of the physician's fee schedule. Thus, if an extender provided a service that would result in a $100 payment to a physician, the payment would be $85. However, there are two important exceptions to this rule. First, if the extender and physician both see the patient during an office visit, the combined work of both the extender and physician is reimbursed at 100 percent of the physician fee schedule. But if the patient service is a procedure (as opposed to a visit) and the work is done primarily by the extender, the 85 percent rule applies. Second, extenders are paid at a 100 percent rate if the service provided is "incident to" a previous visit or service provided by a physician. This provision requires that the physician be physically on-site and that the service provided by the extender be related to a diagnosis made earlier by a physician. Note that "incident to" billing only applies to services provided in offices and clinics as opposed to services provided in hospitals. In effect, these rules mean that the majority of extender billings in offices and clinics is at the 100 percent rate, so average extender reimbursement falls closer to 100 percent than to 85 percent of the physician rate.

The impact of extenders on physician costs and revenues is highly variable. After some acclimation time, which is required for the extender to become fully productive, several financial impacts are realized. First, the physician becomes more productive (sees more patients) because the extender can provide the service for a portion of the visit that is billed by the physician. On average nationwide, this increase in the number of billed visits by the physician is estimated to be 10 to 15 percent. Second, the physician's average reimbursement amount increases because the extender is handling the less complex cases. The national average impact on physician billing amount is estimated at 5 to 10 percent. Finally, the extender can see patients independently and bill for those services. On average, extenders see 10 to 20 percent fewer patients than do physicians. Also, because some of these visits are joint with the physician and billed by the physician, the extender can only bill for the remaining visits, which represent 85 to 90 percent of the visits. Of course, the extent to which these synergies are realized depends on demand (volume). The greater the demand for physician services, the faster an extender can become fully productive and the greater is the impact on physician productivity and reimbursement amounts.

At this point in time, the Practice does not use extenders. However, Dr. Mason believes that extenders can play an important role in many, if not all, of the Practice's clinics. As a start, three clinics have been identified for evaluation: the outpatient surgery pre- and post-op clinic, the internal medicine (family practice) clinic, and the eldercare clinic. Dr. Mason then developed the selected data regarding each clinic's physician staffing, productivity, revenues, and costs (shown in Exhibit 26.1). For example, the outpatient surgery pre- and post-op clinic has 2.5

physician FTEs (full-time equivalents) who handle 7,560 patient visits annually, which generate $842,481 of revenue (collections). Annual compensation for the physician FTEs totals $485,000.

Assume that you have been hired as a consultant by the Practice to look into the use of physician extenders. Specifically, Dr. Mason has asked you to (1) estimate the financial impact of using one physician extender at each of the three clinics and (2) recommend the type of extender that is most appropriate for each setting. **These tasks are not trivial and might require assumptions and information to supplement the data presented in the case.**

As a start, you conclude that the national financial impact data presented earlier must be modified to reflect the actual impact on physician productivity in the three settings. Next, you plan to estimate how many additional visits might be generated at each clinic if one extender is employed. Then, the impact on costs and revenues must be examined. Of course, it might be possible to use an extender to reduce the number of physician FTEs rather than to increase volume. This outcome should be explored if appropriate. Regarding physician extender costs, annual compensation for both NPs and PAs falls into the $80,000 to $100,000 range, depending on geographic location, clinical setting, and work experience.

One of the keys to the analysis is an estimate of the volumes that could be realized at each clinic should an extender be added. Unfortunately, Dr. Mason has only anecdotal evidence (office watercooler speculation) on future demand. The best estimate is that patient volume at the outpatient surgery pre- and post-op clinic is increasing at a 15 percent annual rate as outpatient surgery volume increases. The situation at the internal medicine clinic is quite different. There is a current several-month backlog in scheduling, and hence a physician extender could be fully utilized in a relatively short time. Finally, volume at the eldercare clinic has been sporadic and growing very slowly, so there is some doubt about whether or not another clinician is needed at this time.

Dr. Mason recognizes that you are working with a minimum amount of hard data. Thus, it is important that you express and support the assumptions used in your analysis very clearly.

EXHIBIT 26.1
Shasta Faculty Practice:
Selected Data for Three
Outpatient Clinics

Outpatient Surgery Pre- and Post-Op Clinic:

Physician FTEs	2.5
Physician costs	$485,000
Physician fees (collections)	$842,481
Daily patient utilization	36
Number of days per week	5
Number of weeks per year	42
Annual patient utilization	7,560
Number of visits per physician	3,024

Internal Medicine (Family Practice) Clinic:

Physician FTEs	2.0
Physician costs	$273,500
Physician fees (collections)	$523,290
Daily patient utilization	30
Number of days per week	4
Number of weeks per year	46
Annual patient utilization	5,520
Number of visits per physician	2,760

Eldercare Clinic:

Physician FTEs	2.25
Physician costs	$335,000
Physician fees (collections)	$454,219
Daily patient utilization	23
Number of days per week	4
Number of weeks per year	48
Annual patient utilization	4,416
Number of visits per physician	1,963

Note: Most physicians in the Practice receive compensation from the University in addition to the amounts listed in this exhibit.

JONES MEMORIAL HOSPITAL

27

COMPETING TECHNOLOGIES WITH BACKFILL

JONES MEMORIAL HOSPITAL (the Hospital) is an 800-bed, acute care, not-for-profit teaching hospital affiliated with one of the largest public universities in the United States. In addition to serving the primary and secondary clinical care needs of the neighboring population, the Hospital serves as a tertiary and quaternary referral center for the entire region. For the most part, referred patients seek specialty care that requires unique and often costly clinical expertise and treatment that is available only at select institutions. Thus, it is not surprising that specialty care programs provide the Hospital with about 75 percent of its net operating income.

The Hospital's Center for Digestive Disorders (the Center) is one of the most successful of the specialty care programs. It consistently ranks among the best programs in the country in the diagnosis and treatment of disorders of the gastrointestinal tract. The Center's excellent reputation is further evidenced by the extent of its research funding and its ability to attract patients outside the immediate service area.

The 20 gastroenterologists who staff the Center are physicians drawn from the faculty of the university's College of Medicine. Unlike private practitioners, who focus exclusively on the clinical care of patients, faculty physicians pursue a tripartite mission of clinical service, research, and teaching. It is the successful combination of these pursuits that has helped elevate the status of the Center.

The Center provides care that ranges from gastrointestinal screening to the diagnosis and therapy of common and rare disorders to the referral of appropriate patients to faculty surgeons for the treatment of benign and malignant diseases. The Center encompasses three separate business units: an outpatient clinic, a hospital-based endoscopy suite, and a hospital-based motility (movement) laboratory. Each business unit operates as a separate profit center, and hence each unit maintains its own budget. However, from a patient perspective the care provided is seamless because the Hospital's patient management system expedites patient flow among the Center's three units and to outpatient surgery or inpatient status when required.

Although the motility lab generates less than 5 percent of the Center's total net patient service revenue, it is a vital component. The lab currently performs 600 manometry tests per year. These tests measure the pressure (flow) along the gastrointestinal tract, which assists in the diagnosis of gastrointestinal disorders that cannot be diagnosed visually. The prevalence of disorders such as noncardiac chest pain, dysphasia, gastroesophageal reflux disease, and small bowel motility disorders make manometry testing beneficial to significant segments of the population.

Each test involves the insertion of catheters (probes) into a patient's gastrointestinal tract that relay data back to a computer workstation for analysis. Two technologies are used in motility testing: water perfusion and solid-state. The Center currently has three water perfusion workstations dedicated to motility testing, each of which is used to perform roughly 200 tests per year.

Both water perfusion and solid-state technologies provide relatively reliable data for diagnosis. Furthermore, net reimbursement averages $250 per test regardless of technology, and the current per test operating costs are identical: $150 for labor, $30 for medical supplies, and $15 for administrative supplies.

However, there are distinct differences between the two technologies, the most important of which is patient venue. Water perfusion technology requires the patient to spend one day as an inpatient, while solid-state technology can be done on an outpatient basis. Thus, each test using solid-state rather than water perfusion technology frees up one bed-day for other purposes. In general, the space that is freed up by new projects or technology is called "backfill space," so any beds that would be made available for other purposes by replacing water perfusion with solid-state technology are called "backfill beds."

Although the Center is known for its state-of-the-art technology, its motility laboratory currently has some dated manometry equipment. The Center's medical director, Dr. Carl Forsyth, has made proposals in the past to update the equipment, but more pressing capital investment needs within the Center have kept the proposals from being funded. However, one of the workstations is becoming increasingly unreliable, which has inconvenienced patients and created backlogs. In addition, manometry demand has grown to the point where some patients are being referred to other providers to ensure timely testing. These factors have prompted the Center's administrative director, Edith Hargrove, to seek immediate approval for the acquisition of one new manometry system.

To begin the capital expenditure request process, Edith is currently reviewing quotes from various manufacturers of manometry equipment. Her research on quality and cost has narrowed the field of competing manufacturers to one: Digestive Diagnostics, Inc. A water perfusion workstation, which Edith favors, would cost $25,000, while the nine catheters needed to properly equip the workstation would cost $500 each. The new generation of water perfusion systems, but **not** solid-state systems, has lower per test supply costs: $15 for medical supplies and $10 for administrative supplies.

On the other hand, Dr. Forsyth believes that the Center should purchase a solid-state technology workstation. Regardless of the technology purchased, the existing unreliable water perfusion workstation would be "junked," as it is no longer capable of providing satisfactory service.

Edith, who is a clinically trained nurse, questions the clinical necessity of solid-state technology, especially in light of its higher cost. Although the cost of the workstation is the same ($25,000), the cost of the catheters is substantially higher: $6,000 for each solid-state catheter versus $500 for each water perfusion catheter. Nine catheters are required for both technologies, so the total cost for catheters would be $54,000 for solid-state technology versus only $4,500 for water perfusion technology. In addition, solid-state technology has higher operating (supply) costs than does the new water perfusion technology.

Dr. Forsyth agrees with the capital and operating cost estimates, but he argues that the higher cost of solid-state technology is justified for the following reasons:

1. Solid-state technology enables a technician to perform two tests in the time it takes to do one using water perfusion; rather than performing 200 tests per workstation per year using water perfusion, 400

tests could be performed with solid-state. This would
shorten patient wait time for appointments, decrease
the four-month backlog for motility testing, and
potentially increase overall volume for the Center
from 600 to 800 tests.

2. The current water perfusion technology requires
close observation and correct body positioning during
testing to ensure accurate data collection. As a result,
each patient is kept in a hospital bed as an observation
patient. Conversely, solid-state technology enables
the tests to be performed on an outpatient basis.
This point is of particular interest to the Hospital
because under current operations every test using
water perfusion is a bed-day that cannot be filled by
a medical/surgical patient. Each bed-day for a "true"
inpatient yields an average contribution margin of
$520, whereas the bed-day contribution margin for a
motility test patient is only $40.

3. Solid-state technology is quickly becoming the
standard of care; not offering it would damage the
Center's reputation.

4. Solid-state technology would enhance the teaching
curriculum for residents and fellows and would
provide additional opportunities for research funding.

To his credit, Dr. Forsyth is a respected physician with a reputation
for providing the very best of patient care and at the same time remaining aware of his responsibilities to do so in the most cost-effective way
possible. However, he has been criticized in the past for lobbying Hospital administrators for medical equipment that, in retrospect, could be
considered nothing more than "toys" for himself and his colleagues.

Edith listened to Dr. Forsyth's case for solid-state technology. She
believes he makes some good points, especially in regard to the clinical
efficiencies of solid-state technology. Still, in an environment where
resources are limited and maintaining a positive bottom line is increasingly important, Edith continues to believe that the cost of the solid-
state catheters is a financial burden the lab cannot afford, especially
when reimbursement is the same regardless of the technology used.

The two technology proposals have been brought to the attention
of the Hospital's chief operating officer, Belinda Brach, for resolution.

Believing that a detailed financial analysis is the only rational basis for a decision, she has asked you, a recently hired financial analyst, to investigate the situation. Specifically, she has asked you to use capital budgeting techniques to evaluate the two technologies and make a recommendation on which one to choose.

In addition, Belinda provided some much needed guidance. First, assume that the life of both technologies is five years and that it is unlikely that either the workstations or the catheters would have any salvage value after five years of use. Second, there is no good methodology available to estimate the additional number of tests (more than 200) that might result from pent-up demand if solid-state technology is used. Volume might increase by 100 tests (to 300), but it could increase by as few as 50 or as many as 150. Third, it is very difficult to say how many of the bed-days that are freed up if solid-state technology is used would actually be filled by medical/surgical patients. Again, without good data, she suggests that you assume that 100 additional medical/surgical bed-days would result, but this number could be as low as 80 or as high as 175. Fourth, standard practice calls for all capital-budgeting analyses to assume a 3 percent inflation rate in both costs and reimbursements. Finally, the Hospital's corporate cost of capital is 10 percent, and it adds or subtracts 3 percentage points to account for differential risk.

Just as you were about to start the analysis, the phone rang; it was Belinda. She said it was likely that she could put her hands on some additional funding to buy a second system, but the amount would only be enough to buy a water perfusion system. When you asked Edith what the lab would do with the second system—if it, too, should be replaced—she said the Hospital could sell it for about $10,000 because it was only three years old. Edith added, "You might as well crunch the numbers on the potential second system while you're at it."

*Working
Capital*

FOSTER PHARMACEUTICALS

RECEIVABLES MANAGEMENT

28

Kathleen Grogan received her PhD in pharmacology ten years ago from Boston University. While there, she became very interested in the business side of drug distribution and hence stayed on for an extra 18 months to earn an MBA. After graduation, she went to work for Capo Corporation, a major drug manufacturer, where she managed the development of a new nonprescription antiallergy drug. Although the drug passed all Food and Drug Administration (FDA) trials and was certified for general use, Capo simultaneously developed a similar drug that was cheaper to produce and equally effective in treating most, but not all, allergy symptoms. Thus, Capo decided not to proceed with production of the drug that Kathleen helped develop. However, Capo was willing to license production and distribution rights to another company. Kathleen thought that this might be a golden opportunity, so she quit her job with Capo to found her own company, Foster Pharmaceuticals. The sole purpose of the new company is to obtain the license for, produce, and distribute the new drug, which Kathleen dubbed "SneezeRelief."

Kathleen is currently working on the business plan that she will present at a venture capital conference to be held in New York. The main purpose of the conference is to match entrepreneurs with venture capitalists who are interested in providing capital to fledgling firms. Kathleen has spent a lot of time thinking about how her proposed company's receivables should be managed; she is concerned about this issue because she knows of several small drug manufacturers that

193

have gotten into serious financial difficulty because of poor receivables management.

Initially, Foster Pharmaceuticals would sell directly and exclusively to four retail customers in the Northeast (Exhibit 28.1 provides the sales mix). If demand proved solid, the company would expand into other areas and wholesale channels. Sales are expected to be highly seasonal: Allergy drug sales are slow during the winter months, but they pick up dramatically in the spring when plant pollen levels reach a peak. Business falls off again in the summer, but it picks up in the fall when the ragweed season begins. Kathleen's sales forecasts for the first six months of operations are given in Exhibit 28.2. Assuming the fledgling company receives financing and begins operations, Kathleen's sales forecasts for the first six months of the second year are provided in Exhibit 28.3.

Kathleen does not plan to give discounts for early payment; discounts are not widely used in the industry. Based on preliminary discussions with the retail outlets (her customers) Kathleen forecasts the payment schedule, shown in Exhibit 28.4. She does not foresee any problems with bad-debt losses; the retailers she plans to sell to have been in business for a long time. Furthermore, she plans to carefully screen her customers, and she believes that these two factors will eliminate such losses. On average, Kathleen believes that 20 percent of receivables will contribute to profits, so 80 percent of receivables represent cash costs. Furthermore, the First National Bank of New England has indicated that its receivables financing would cost 8 percent annually.

In spite of her optimism regarding bad-debt losses, Kathleen is concerned about the company's potential level of receivables, and she wants to have a monitoring system in place that will allow her to quickly spot any adverse trends that develop. Kathleen's total sales forecast for the first full year of operations is 800,000 packages. Each package, which will contain 12 tablets, will be priced at $5.

Kathleen has hired you as an outside consultant to advise her about receivables management. So far, you have developed a model that produces accounts receivable balances, average collection period (ACP), aging schedules, uncollected balances schedules, and quarterly carrying costs for the end of March and the end of June. The uncollected balances schedule permits managers to remove the effects of seasonal and/or cyclical sales variation and to construct an accurate measure of receivables payment patterns. Thus, it provides financial managers with better aggregate information than do such crude measures as the ACP or aging schedule.

Kathleen anticipates that the venture capitalists will ask some questions concerning the interpretation of the receivables data, the sensitivity of the results to the basic assumptions, and strategies to reduce carrying costs of receivables.

Customer	Sales Mix
Large retail chain 1	40%
Large retail chain 2	35%
Regional drug store	15%
Small grocery chain	10%

EXHIBIT 28.1
Foster Pharmaceuticals: Forecast Customer Sales Mix

Month	Sales
January	$100,000
February	250,000
March	400,000
April	600,000
May	450,000
June	300,000

EXHIBIT 28.2
Foster Pharmaceuticals: Partial Sales Forecasts for Year 1

Month	Sales
January	$200,000
February	350,000
March	500,000
April	700,000
May	550,000
June	350,000

EXHIBIT 28.3
Foster Pharmaceuticals: Partial Sales Forecasts for Year 2

EXHIBIT 28.4
Foster Pharmaceuticals:
Forecast Receivables
Collection Pattern

Customer	0–30 Days	31–60 Days	61–90 Days
Large retail chain 1	35%	50%	15%
Large retail chain 2	25%	40%	35%
Regional drug store	20%	35%	45%
Small grocery chain	30%	55%	15%

CLARINDA COMMUNITY HOSPITAL
INVENTORY MANAGEMENT

29

CLARINDA COMMUNITY HOSPITAL is a 230-bed, not-for-profit, acute care hospital located in Clarinda, Iowa. The city is a typical Midwestern county seat/farming community best known as the birthplace of Glenn Miller, the famous big band leader of the late 1930s and early 1940s.

The hospital carries more than 10,000 different items of inventory that vary widely in price, order lead times, and stockout costs. (Stockout costs are the total costs that result from running out of stock of a particular inventory item, including higher costs of service caused by scheduling delays or emergency replenishments as well as the costs associated with negative patient outcomes and potential lawsuits.)

Clarinda uses the ABC method of inventory classification, also called selective inventory control, along with a variety of inventory-control methods, to manage its different inventory items. The ABC classification system works in this way: Clarinda maintains data on the average annual usage and unit cost of each inventory item, which typically is called a stock-keeping unit (SKU). Then, the dollar usage (Average annual usage × Unit cost) is calculated for each SKU. Next, these amounts are converted into percentages of total dollar usage and the SKUs are arrayed from highest to lowest percentage. The SKUs are then divided into three groups (or classes), labeled A, B, and C, using the general guidelines provided in Exhibit 29.1.

To better utilize the limited resources available for inventory management, Clarinda's managers focus most of their attention on Class A items. The usage rates, stock positions, and delivery times for SKUs in this class are reviewed on a biweekly basis, with control and ordering system data adjusted as necessary. Class B items are reviewed every quarter, while Class C items are reviewed semiannually.

Even though this process has served Clarinda well, Marco Muñoz, the hospital's newly hired chief financial officer, thinks the hospital is carrying excess inventories. He notes that Clarinda has never come close to having a stockout, even when it has been running near 100 percent occupancy. Marco believes that a thorough review should be undertaken of all Class A items and that it might be possible to increase inventory turnover by 25 percent, and hence lower inventory carrying costs, by trimming current stocks.

To convince Clarinda's CEO, Marco plans to perform a demonstration inventory analysis that focuses on the forms used by the surgical intensive care unit (SICU). Different forms are required for almost every aspect of SICU operations, including records of patient progress; requests for lab tests, blood products, and medications; nurse and physician notes; and transfer/discharge instructions. Exhibit 29.2 shows inventory usage and cost data on the SICU's 25 forms. To begin his demonstration analysis, Marco plans to conduct a new ABC analysis on the SICU's inventory. (Clarinda is in the process of converting to computerized forms as part of the transition to electronic medical records, but the paper forms will still be used for several years.)

As part of its commitment to supporting the local economy, Clarinda currently uses a single local source for all of the SICU's forms: Atwood Printing and Office Supplies (Supplier A). Supplier A requires a $25 set-up fee on each order, in addition to the cost per unit. Clarinda is considering using a national supplier, Bateman Medical Office Products (Supplier B), which charges no set-up fee but does charge $50 to cover postage and handling. Supplier B takes three days to deliver the forms, versus only one day for Supplier A. Processing each order will cost Clarinda another $25, regardless of which supplier is used. Thus, the total order cost is $50 for Supplier A and $75 for Supplier B.

Marco's ultimate goal is to use economic ordering quantity (EOQ) concepts to select the supplier for all forms used by the SICU. His primary areas of concern are (1) the number of orders placed each year, (2) reorder points (in units), and (3) total inventory costs. As part of the demonstration analysis, Marco will focus on the form used to order blood products from the hospital's blood bank (SKU number 53104 in Exhibit 29.2). The data associated with Suppliers A and B, as well as inventory carrying costs and other data, are summarized in Exhibit 29.3.

In addition to an analysis without safety stocks, Marco is concerned about the impact of safety stocks on the decision. Clarinda currently carries a safety stock of two units of SKU 53104 to protect itself against stockouts as a result of delivery delays and/or an increase in the usage rate. When asked how that amount was arrived at, the manager of the SICU stated that she didn't know and that they had always done it that way. However, if the hospital decides to switch to Supplier B, the manager stated that it seems logical to increase the safety stock to six units to reflect Supplier B's three-times-as-long lead time. Of particular interest are the impact of safety stocks on inventory costs, the safety margins that such stocks would provide against higher-than-expected usage and shipping delays, and whether or not the current lead time for Supplier A and the estimate for Supplier B make any sense.

Also, Marco has heard a rumor that Supplier B is about to offer a 10 percent discount if the entire year's demand (92 units) is ordered at once. He wants to know what the impact of this discount would be on the decision about which supplier to use. Also, it would be useful to know how high a discount is needed to make Supplier B less costly than Supplier A.

Furthermore, Marco knows that it is unlikely that the forms would be ordered exactly as prescribed by the EOQ model, so he would like to know the impact of ordering variations on total inventory costs. Finally, Marco knows that Clarinda's CEO has expressed some doubt about the value of the EOQ model in making real-world inventory decisions. "If I'm right in my concerns," he asked, "what other inventory control methods are available to us?"

Place yourself in Marco's shoes and see if you can conduct the demonstration analysis that he has in mind.

**EXHIBIT 29.1
ABC Classification
Guidance**

Classification	Inventory Value	Inventory Amount
A	60–70%	10–20%
B	20–30%	30–40%
C	10–20%	50–60%

**EXHIBIT 29.2
Clarinda Community
Hospital: Form Inventory
Data for SICU**

SKU Number	Unit Size	Supplier A Unit Cost	Units Used Annually
50071	25	$ 31	3
50083	25	16	4
50084	50	18	14
50091	250	86	28
50100	25	22	4
50102	250	793	3
50122	250	196	2
50129	250	177	3
50131	100	122	5
50132	100	98	5
50138	100	26	9
50139	50	21	10
50170	100	8	83
50172	100	44	4
50174	500	62	8
50193	25	2	66
50194	100	122	2
50206	250	11	279
50472	100	192	2
50475	125	551	4
50694	100	18	10
51060	100	102	6
53006	50	17	4
53104	50	66	92
57134	100	16	5

Expected annual usage	92 units
Cost per Unit:	
Supplier A	$66
Supplier B	$60
Inventory Carrying Costs:	
Depreciation	0.0%
Storage and handling	17.1
Interest expense	6.6
Property taxes	0.4
Insurance	0.9
Total carrying costs	25.0%
Inventory Ordering Costs:	
Supplier A	$50
Supplier B	$75
Current Safety Stocks:	
Supplier A	2 units
Supplier B (estimate)	6 units
Delivery Times:	
Supplier A	1 day
Supplier B	3 days

**EXHIBIT 29.3
Clarinda Community
Hospital Cost and
Usage Data: Blood
Product Ordering Form
(SKU 53104)**

MILWAUKEE REGIONAL HEALTH SYSTEM

REVENUE CYCLE MANAGEMENT

30

Andrew Mae has recently been hired as the vice president of Revenue Cycle Management for the Milwaukee Regional Health System (MRHS), an integrated system with approximately $2.5 billion in annual revenues. Located in the Milwaukee metropolitan area, MRHS consists of an academic medical center, two community hospitals, and 30 outpatient primary and specialty care clinics. Annually, the hospitals collectively see more than 40,000 admissions, approximately 100,000 emergency room visits, and nearly 1 million outpatient encounters, while the clinics receive more than 1.6 million visits.

The vice president of Revenue Cycle Management is a newly created position at MRHS. In that role, Andrew will oversee the merger of the currently separate hospital and physician revenue cycle departments. Andrew has been directed by MRHS's CEO to accomplish two primary goals: (1) lower the overall costs of revenue cycle management and (2) improve the revenue cycle process. (For more information on revenue cycle management, see the Healthcare Financial Management Association website at www.hfma.org or the Medical Group Management Association website at www.mgma.com. Search the term *revenue cycle* at either or both websites.)

Andrew understands that the first step in merging MRHS's separate revenue cycle departments is to alter the current perception that hospital and physician practice revenue cycles are inherently different. His goal in this regard is to illustrate the similarities between and interdependencies among the revenue cycle processes to highlight what he believes to be the true determinants of revenue cycle success: (1) the collective hospital, physician, and revenue cycle staffs' effort to limit defects in the process and (2) the ability to identify, bill, and collect the correct net realizable value of each encounter. When asked about these statements, Andrew explained that defects can be thought of as problems that impede the revenue cycle process, while net realizable value is the actual dollar amount expected to be collected from both patient and insurer for each service provided.

To begin the effort, Andrew prepared an orientation presentation for hospital and physician leadership on the integrated revenue cycle management process. Following is part of that presentation:

The revenue cycle management process in healthcare provider organizations represents the process of identifying and securing the financial integrity of all services and care provided by the organization. It encompasses the information systems, policies, and methodologies used by an organization to review patients' and insurers' financial responsibilities, document the services and care provided, translate those activities to the appropriate billing amounts, issue invoices, and collect the correct payments. The revenue cycle management process also includes the evaluation of receivables (outstanding balances due for services provided) and the continuous review of the contract and auditing functions to ensure that all actions are in compliance with MRHS's hundreds of third-party payer contracts.

The schematic shown below presents an overview of a typical provider revenue cycle management process as described by the Medical Group Management Association. It is followed by a brief description of each

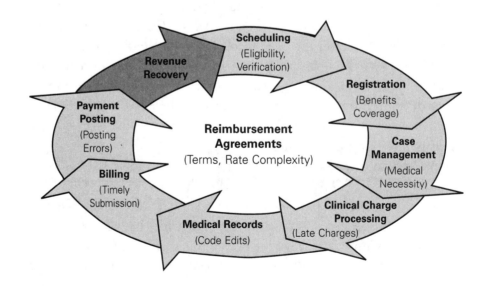

function and the information gathered within the function, beginning with the scheduling function, which typically begins the revenue cycle process. Some potential defects that can occur within each function are also listed. It is important to understand that immediate identification and correction of defects are critical to good revenue cycle performance because they can create bottlenecks, require reprocessing, result in poor patient experiences, and/or reduce net realizable values.

Scheduling. Typically, this function is the first interaction between the patient and the provider system. Hence, scheduling represents the beginning of the revenue cycle process.

- Scheduling occurs throughout the hospital and clinic settings; emergency department and walk-in patients require unique scheduling procedures.
- Patient information gathering begins with the description of the health issue/care need and type of insurance coverage.
- Examples of potential defects during the execution of this function include directing patients to the wrong service and failing to properly identify and verify insurance coverage and obtain precertification (if required).

Registration. This is the first patient experience on the first day of each patient encounter.

- Registration occurs throughout the hospital and clinic settings.
- Patient information gathered in the scheduling process is confirmed or updated, and additional health condition and financial/insurance information is obtained if needed.
- Examples of potential defects during the execution of this function include misidentifying patient and/or insurer information and failing to verify coverage and precertification (if required).

Case management. With this function, the translation of medically necessary healthcare services to charges for those services begins.

- Case management occurs throughout the hospital and clinic settings, with a particular emphasis on hospital inpatient admissions.
- Patients' medical history and documentation of current status and care plan are reviewed.
- Examples of potential defects during the execution of this function include ordering and/or performing services that are not preauthorized or are deemed medically unnecessary by the insurer.

Clinical charge processing. Here, the clinical documentation of services provided is translated to line-item charges.

- Clinical charge processing, which applies to hospital and clinic services, uses diagnosis-related group (DRG) and revenue codes for hospital billing and Current Procedural Terminology (CPT) and Healthcare Common Procedure Coding System codes for outpatient and physician billing.
- Documentation of all services and the level of care provided is matched to the charge description master (chargemaster) file.
- Examples of potential defects during the execution of this function include charges submitted after the allowed documentation period (late charges) and improper matching of clinical entries with the chargemaster file.

Medical records. This function consists of the systematic compilation and documentation of all care provided to patients during and, if appropriate, subsequent to the encounter.

- A single patient record for all services is created.
- Information in the record is available to patients and other care providers, subject to certain regulations and restrictions.
- Examples of potential defects during the execution of this function include documentation and coding errors and lag times in the coding and compiling of the record (discharged but not billed).

Billing. This function converts the information gathered in previous functions to patient and insurer bills (invoices).

- In the billing function, UB04 forms (for hospital inpatient and outpatient insurance billing) and CMS 1500 forms (for physician insurance billing) are prepared.
- Given the highly technical nature of the UB04 and CMS 1500 forms, separate billing statements are created for patients that indicate their payment responsibilities.
- Examples of potential defects during the execution of this function include a lack of timely bill submission and failure to follow the specific billing rules required by the insurer, which results in payment denials.

Payment posting. In this function, the accounts receivable entry is adjusted as invoices are collected. Note that this process may require a coordinated effort of follow-up and collections actions directed at the insurer and/or patient.

- Payment posting is complicated by the many different rules, regulations, and data formats required by private and government insurers.
- Unpaid balances due from patients undergo another round of processing, including research to find additional insurance and/or financial status information.
- Examples of potential defects during the execution of this function include mishandling of insurer payment denials, posting errors that misstate the remaining outstanding balance from patients, and patients' confusion over insurer invoicing and coverage.

Revenue recovery. This audit function takes place continuously to examine the entire revenue cycle process. The following steps are taken during revenue recovery:

- Measure the performance of each revenue cycle function according to established benchmarks.
- Identify the cause of each defect and take corrective action as necessary.
- Ensure compliance with regulatory requirements and confirm that payments received are consistent with all insurer contract provisions and the organization's charity care policy.
- Defects that can occur in this function include improper selection of benchmark metrics and/or values and failure to aggressively audit and/or correct defects in the revenue cycle.

The hospital and physician leaders found Andrew's presentation to be a valuable overview of the revenue cycle process. However, they remained concerned over the merging of the two revenue cycle departments and questioned the metrics chosen to monitor performance. In addition, they expressed a need to know more about the concept of defects and how to identify and correct them. Finally, the leaders wanted to learn more about net realizable value, specifically, the differences across the most important insurer contracts. To address these issues, Andrew began to create two documents: one that includes both hospital and clinic revenue cycle performance metrics and another that highlights the differences in reimbursement methodologies and net realizable values. **Note that all metric and reimbursement values provided in this case are for instructional use only and should not be used for other purposes.**

The next meeting with hospital and physician leadership is scheduled in two weeks, and Andrew had planned to complete the two projects prior to the meeting. Unfortunately, Andrew broke his leg in a snowmobile accident and requires surgery and a short hospitalization, so he is unable to get the work done in time for the meeting. Thus, he has asked you, an administrative fellow at MRHS, to help out. He has given you the following three tasks:

1. Establish two overall revenue cycle performance metrics and one defect metric for each revenue cycle function, from scheduling through payment posting. The metrics should be based on nationally accepted practices, and the list should include definitions and current benchmark values. Andrew has already started this task, so he provided you with the template shown in Exhibit 30.1, which contains one overall performance metric, accounts receivable (A/R) days, already filled in. Also, he finished compiling a list of metric candidates and benchmark values from various sources, which is provided in Exhibit 30.2. Thus, your task is to choose one additional overall performance metric and the single best defect metric for each function listed in Exhibit 30.1 for both the hospital and clinic settings. Andrew mentioned that there will be a great deal of discussion of these metrics at the meeting, so it is essential that you fully justify your selections.

2. Compare the MRHS actual values for the metrics chosen, provided in Exhibit 30.3, with the benchmark values. Discuss the implications of your comparisons and, most important, suggest the corrective actions that should be implemented to bring MRHS in line with national standards for the areas of subpar performance.

3. Every year, MRHS performs an extensive pricing study comparing its gross charges (chargemaster prices) to other healthcare providers in its market in order to competitively align its price structure. Of course, MRHS typically gets paid far less than gross charges for the care it provides. The actual billing amount is determined by analyzing the hundreds of reimbursement contracts the system has in force with

insurers as well as policies that MRHS has in place for indigent patients. (For more information about chargemaster pricing, refer to "The Pricing of U.S. Hospital Services: Chaos Behind a Veil of Secrecy," by Uwe E. Reinhardt, posted at http://content. healthaffairs.org/content/25/1/57.full.) Andrew wants to highlight the role that contract provisions with insurers play in determining the final reimbursement amount. Thus, Andrew has asked you to calculate the expected total reimbursement amount according to gross (chargemaster) prices, the reimbursement model used, and the actual collections experience for two common procedures: CPT 73722 (MRI of the knee) and DRG 470 (major joint replacement). To help you, Andrew has created the following template, with one cell completed. After you finish the table, Andrew would like you to assess the fairness and efficiency of the current fragmented payment system to providers, insurers, patients, and society (the ultimate bearers of healthcare costs). In addition, you have been asked to calculate the average expected payment for the MRI and joint replacement procedures. (MRHS's payer mix is 46 percent Medicare, 34 percent commercial/ managed care, 16 percent Medicaid, and 4 percent self-pay/no insurance.)

	MRI of the Knee CPT 73722 Charge = $2,800	Major Joint Replacement (4-day LOS) DRG 470 Charge = $50,000
Medicare		
Base payment rate	$341.61	$17,955.00
No-payment denial rate of 3%	(10.25)	
Part A deductible of $1,184 @ 65% collection rate	N/A	
Part B deductible of $140 @ 78% collection rate	(30.80)	
Total reimbursement	**$300.56**	
Medicaid		
Per diem of $284/visit or $2,044/day		
No-payment denial rate of 0.5%		
Total reimbursement		
Commercial/Managed Care		
58% of charge		
No-payment denial rate of 12%		
20% patient coinsurance @ 40% collection rate		
Total reimbursement		
Self-Pay/No Insurance		
30% discount		
5% self-pay collection rate		
Total reimbursement		

Hint: All of the data needed to complete this table are listed on the template labels. Note that the chargemaster price for each procedure and the length of stay (LOS) for the joint replacement are listed in the column header information. Also, remember that Medicare Part A pays for inpatient services (joint replacement), while Part B pays for outpatient services (MRI).

	Metric	Metric Definition	Hospital Benchmark	Clinic Benchmark
Overall Metrics	A/R days	Net patient accounts receivable/(Annual patient service revenue/365 days)	48.3 days	28.5 days
Defect Metrics				
Scheduling				
Registration				
Case management				
Clinical charge processing				
Medical records				
Billing				
Payment posting				

EXHIBIT 30.1
Benchmarking Template

EXHIBIT 30.2
Selected National
Benchmark Data

	Metric Definition	Hospital Benchmark	Clinic Benchmark
Overall Metrics			
A/R days	Net patient accounts receivable/ (Annual net patient revenue/365 days)	48.3 days	28.5 days
Percent of A/R greater than 90 days	Accounts receivable aged greater than 90 days/Total accounts receivable	29.6%	19.0%
Cost to collect	Total revenue cycle costs/ Total cash collected	3.5%	4.2%
Defect Metrics			
Scheduling			
Preregistration rate	No. of patient encounters preregistered/ No. of scheduled patient encounters	84.8%	99.1%
Insurance verification rate	No. of verified encounters/ No. of registered encounters	90.0%	98.7%
Registration			
Point-of-service collection rate	Point-of-service cash collections/ Total patient cash collected	13.4%	36.2%
Registration quality score	No. of correct patient demographic and insurance data elements input/ Total data elements required at registration	98.7%	99.4%
Case management			
Preauthorization denial rate	No. of claims denied for no preauth/ No. of claims submitted	1.8%	0.7%
Percent of medical necessity write-offs	Medical necessity write-offs/Total charges	0.4%	0.6%
Clinical charge processing			
Charge lag days	Days between service date and posting of charge/Encounters billed	3.6 days	5.1 days
Late charge %	Charges posted more than 3 days after the date of service/Total charges	8.4%	78.6%

	Metric Definition	Hospital Benchmark	Clinic Benchmark
Medical records			
Days in total discharged not final billed	Gross dollars in accounts receivable unbilled/(Annual net patient revenue/ 365 days)	7.4 days	5.9 days
Coding quality score	No. of correct coding data elements input/ Total data elements required at coding	96.5%	93.2%
Billing			
Initial denial rate	No. of claims denied/No. of claims submitted	4.9%	8.2%
Clean claim rate	No. of claims that pass edits with no manual intervention/Total billed claims	76.8%	81.2%
Payment posting			
Percent of payments posted electronically	Dollars posted electronically/ Total payments posted	86.7%	83.1%
Net days revenue in credit balance*	Dollars in credit balance/ (Annual net patient revenue/365 days)	1.9 days	3.2 days

*Credit balance reflects monies owed to payers due to improper billing.

EXHIBIT 30.2 (continued) Selected National Benchmark Data

EXHIBIT 30.3
Selected MRHS
Metric Values

	MRHS Hospitals	MRHS Clinics
Overall Metrics		
A/R days	45.4 days	26.3 days
% of A/R greater than 90 days	21.5%	20.1%
Cost to collect	2.9%	4.5%
Defect Metrics		
Scheduling		
Preregistration rate	80.8%	99.9%
Insurance verification rate	85.3%	100.0%
Registration		
Point-of-service collection rate	8.7%	48.5%
Registration quality score	91.6%	99.9%
Case management		
Preauthorization denial rate	2.4%	0.3%
Percent of medical necessity write-offs	0.7%	0.2%
Clinical charge processing		
Charge lag days	3.2 days	6.8 days
Late charge percent	2.1%	86.9%
Medical records		
Days in total discharged not final billed	4.5 days	7.5 days
Coding quality score	98.7%	90.2%
Billing		
Initial denial rate	5.6%	7.8%
Clean claim rate	72.4%	85.2%
Payment posting		
Percent of payments posted electronically	90.1%	78.9%
Net days revenue in credit balance	2.5 days	2.3 days

Other Topics

RIVER COMMUNITY HOSPITAL (B)

FINANCIAL FORECASTING

31

RIVER COMMUNITY HOSPITAL is a 210-bed, not-for-profit, acute care hospital with a long-standing reputation for quality service to a growing service area. River competes with three other hospitals in its metropolitan statistical area (MSA): two not-for-profit and one for-profit. It is the smallest of the four but has traditionally been ranked highest in patient satisfaction polls. For a complete description of the hospital, along with its 2011–2013 financial statements, see Case 1: River Community Hospital (A).

As the newly hired special assistant to the CEO, you have completed the financial and operating analyses (see Case 1) assigned by your boss, Melissa Randolph. In fact, your presentation to the board of trustees went so well that Melissa asked you to present the hospital's preliminary five-year financial plan at the next board meeting. To aid in the planning process, she provided the following information:

1. Given your knowledge of the historical situation for River, current trends in the healthcare industry, and the competitive situation facing hospitals today, use your own best judgment to create the hospital's financial plan. Make any assumptions you believe to be necessary to create the plan, including assumptions about inpatient and outpatient volume growth, capacity constraints, reimbursement patterns, hospital staffing patterns, input cost inflation, and so on. Be sure to completely document your assumptions in the

217

report. **You have very limited specific information about the hospital, so use your general knowledge about trends in the hospital industry to make the forecasts. The quality of your financial plan will be judged as much (or more) on the validity of your assumptions as on the mechanics of the forecasting process.**

2. The emphasis should be on the forecast for the first year (2014), but you should also create rough income statements, balance sheets, and statements of cash flows for the following four years (five years in total), including key financial ratios.

3. The five primary methods for forecasting income statement items and balance sheet accounts are (a) percentage of sales (in which a constant growth rate is applied), (b) simple linear regression, (c) curvilinear regression, (d) multiple regression, and (e) specific item forecasting. You may need to use several of these methods in your forecast. (Hint: Do not forget that spreadsheets have a regression capability.)

4. Use the financial analysis from Case 1 to help with the forecast if that case was assigned. Those areas where hospital performance has been poor should be improved, and your forecasts should reflect anticipated operational improvements where applicable.

5. Do not get so involved in the mechanics of the forecasting process that you forget to apply common sense to your forecasts. Think about what has happened in the past and what is likely to happen in the future in regard to utilization, prices, costs, and asset requirements. If the forecast does not make sense, modify it until it does. For example, a blind application of statistical forecasting techniques might lead to a forecast containing five years of net operating losses. Regardless of statistical "fit," such a forecast makes no sense because any hospital, if it expects to survive, will have to take actions to change utilization, pricing, or cost trends to ensure positive operating results. Thus, the "blindly" forecasted values do not represent what is likely to happen in the future, even

though they might be a perfect reflection of historical trends. Similarly, a forecast that is wildly optimistic probably needs to be modified because payers and competitors likely would react to dampen profitability if it rose dramatically.

In closing, Melissa gave you her view of a good financial plan: "First and foremost, the plan should consist of pro forma financial statements along with a table that summarizes the amount of financing generated internally and any external financing requirements. Second, key financial ratios should be calculated, and the hospital's expected future financial condition should be assessed, with special emphasis on changes from the hospital's current condition. Third, make sure that your forecasted financial statements are consistent with one another. The last special assistant could not figure out that two balance sheet accounts—equity (fund) capital and accumulated depreciation—are tied to income statement items, so he did not last very long. Finally, make all your assumptions clear, and be prepared to answer questions from the board concerning the impact of changes in your assumptions on the financial plan."

SANTA FE HEALTHCARE

CAPITATION AND RISK SHARING

32

SANTA FE MEMORIAL HOSPITAL is a community hospital in Green Bay, Wisconsin. Recently, the hospital and its affiliated physicians formed Santa Fe Healthcare, a physician–hospital organization (the PHO). The PHO is close to signing its first contract to provide exclusive local healthcare services to enrollees in BadgerCare (the Plan), the local Blue Cross Blue Shield of Wisconsin HMO. For the past several years, the Plan has contracted with a different Green Bay PHO, but financial difficulties at that organization have prompted the Plan to consider Santa Fe Healthcare as an alternative. In the proposed contract, the PHO will assume full risk for patient utilization. In fact, the proposal calls for the PHO to receive a fixed premium of $200 per member per month from the Plan, which it then can allocate to each provider component in any way it deems best using any reimbursement method it chooses.

The PHO's executive director, Dr. George O'Donnell, a cardiologist and recent graduate of the University of Wisconsin's Nonresident Program in Administrative Medicine, is evaluating the Plan's proposal. To help do this, Dr. O'Donnell hired a consulting firm that specializes in PHO contracting.

The first task of the consulting firm was to review the PHO's current medical panel and estimate the number of physicians, by specialty, required to support the Plan's patient population of 50,000, assuming aggressive utilization management. The results in Exhibit 32.1 show that the PHO's medical panel currently consists of 249 physicians, while the number of physicians required to support the Plan's patient population

221

is only 59. Note, however, that the PHO physicians serve patients other than those in the Plan, so the total number of physicians required to treat all of the PHO's patients far exceeds the 59 shown in the right column of the exhibit.

The second task of the consulting firm was to analyze the PHO physicians' current practice patterns. It is clear that utilization, and hence cost, is driven by the PHO's physicians and that variation in practice patterns is costly to the PHO. Results of the analysis show significant variation in practice patterns, both in the physicians' offices and in the hospital. For example, Exhibit 32.2 contains summary data on hospital costs by physician for three common diagnosis-related groups (DRGs). Consider DRG 127 (heart failure). The physician with the lowest hospital costs averaged $4,271 in costs per patient, the highest-cost physician averaged $7,394, and the average cost for all physicians was $5,319. The consulting firm commented that it is important to reduce this variation because the PHO is at full risk for patient utilization.

The third task of the consulting firm was to recommend an appropriate allocation of the premium dollars to each category of provider. Specifically, the contract calls for the PHO to receive $200 per member per month, for a total annual revenue of $200 × 50,000 members × 12 months = $120 million. To reduce potential conflicts about how to divide the $120 million among providers, the consulting firm proposed a "status quo" allocation that would maintain the current revenue distribution percentages shown in Exhibit 32.3.

The final task of the consulting firm was to recommend provider reimbursement methodologies that create appropriate incentives. In the contract, the PHO assumes full risk for patient utilization, so the consulting firm recommended that all component providers be capitated to align cost minimization incentives across the entire PHO. Furthermore, capitation of all providers would eliminate the need for risk pools, a risk-sharing arrangement that the PHO has never used. In addition to the consulting firm's report, Dr. O'Donnell decided to ask a new PHO operations committee for a short report on the current status of the major PHO providers. The committee provided him with the following information.

Santa Fe Memorial Hospital

Historically the profitability of Santa Fe Memorial Hospital has been roughly in line with the industry. Last year, when the hospital received about 75 percent of charges, on average, the hospital achieved an operating margin of about 3 percent. However, hospital managers are concerned about its profitability if the Plan's proposal is accepted. The managers believe that the full-risk contract would require extraordinary efforts to control costs and that the most effective way to do this would be to create a subpanel of physicians for participation in the capitation contract. When asked how the subpanel should be chosen, its recommendation was to choose the physicians who would do the best job of containing hospital costs.

Primary Care Physicians

Many of the primary care physicians are dissatisfied. On average, primary care physicians receive only about 60 percent of charges, and they are concerned that they could be penalized by accepting utilization risk for the Plan's enrollees. Primary care physicians know that they are paid less and believe that they have to work much harder than do the specialists. Furthermore, primary care physicians believe that the specialists supplement their own incomes by overusing in-office tests and procedures. Some primary care physicians are even talking about dropping out of the PHO, forming their own contracting group, and taking the whole capitation payment from the Plan and contracting themselves for specialist and hospital services.

Specialist Care Physicians

The specialists believe that the primary care physicians refer too many patients to them. The specialists do not mind the referrals as long as their reimbursement is based on charges because, on average, they receive 90 percent of charges. However, if they are capitated, the specialists want the primary care physicians to handle more of the minor patient problems themselves. Also, whenever the subject of subpanels is raised, many of the specialists become incensed. "After all," they say, "the whole idea behind the PHO is to protect the specialists." Both sets of physicians—primary care and specialist—agree that the hospital is hopelessly inefficient. Said one specialist, "No matter how much revenue the hospital receives, it still seems to barely make a profit."

To respond to the Plan's proposal, Dr. O'Donnell and the PHO's executive committee must decide whether to accept the recommendations of the consulting firm.

Assume that you have been hired to advise Dr. O'Donnell and the executive committee of Santa Fe Healthcare regarding its plan to address these challenges. Your report should address the concerns raised by the physicians and the hospital. Furthermore, the report must provide specific recommendations on how to implement these changes because the report will form the basis for an implementation plan if the contract is accepted.

EXHIBIT 32.1
Santa Fe Healthcare:
Physician PHO Members
and Estimated Needs for
50,000 Enrollees

Specialty	Number in PHO	Estimated Need per 50,000 Enrollees
General medicine	42	20.9
Pediatrics	15	4.1
Total primary care	57	25.0
Anesthesiology	9	2.5
Cardiology	12	1.4
Emergency medicine	10	2.5
General surgery	13	2.7
Neurosurgery	3	0.3
Obstetrics/gynecology	27	5.4
Orthopedics	11	2.5
Psychiatry	19	1.9
Radiology	8	3.0
Thoracic surgery	0	0.4
Urology	5	1.3
Other specialties	75	10.1
Total specialists	192	34.0
Grand total	249	59.0

DRG		Minimum	Average	Maximum
98:	Bronchitis/asthma	$2,872	$4,018	$4,638
127:	Heart failure	4,271	5,319	7,394
373:	Vaginal delivery without complications	6,498	7,568	8,015

Note: This exhibit is based on historical costs related to the old severity-unadjusted DRGs. In the future, the cost data will be related to the new severity-adjusted Medicare severity diagnosis-related groups (MS-DRGs).

EXHIBIT 32.2 Hospital Costs for Three Common DRGs by Physician

PHO administration/overhead	13%
Paid to within-system physicians	
Primary care	10
Specialists	18
Ancillary services	5
Administration/profit	1
Paid to within-system hospital	38
Paid for prescription drugs	10
Paid to out-of-system providers	5
Total premium dollar	100%

EXHIBIT 32.3 Proposed Allocation of Premium Dollars

Ethics
Mini-Cases

TRIGON BLUE CROSS/ BLUE SHIELD

COPAYMENTS

1

WHEN MOST PEOPLE are told they owe a coinsurance payment on a medical bill, they simply grimace and write a check—but not Gerald Haeckel, a retiree from Richmond, Virginia. He wanted proof that he was not paying more than the 20 percent portion that his health insurance policy required. When his insurer, Trigon Blue Cross/Blue Shield, balked, the retiree besieged state and federal officials with demands for an investigation.

Gerald's problem with insurer–provider negotiated discounts began when he became confused by a bill sent by Trigon Blue Cross/Blue Shield. The bill was for Gerald's wife's lumpectomy, which is an outpatient surgery to remove a tiny breast tumor. Trigon's patient benefits statement indicated that the surgery had cost $950, that Trigon paid 80 percent or $760, and that Gerald owed a 20 percent copayment of $190. But then Gerald received a statement of charges and allowances from the surgery center indicating that Trigon's share of the bill had been more than halved to $374 because of a "contractual adjustment." Gerald assumed that a mistake was made in the surgery center's statement, because if it were correct, his $190 copayment would exceed a third of the actual cost, instead of the 20 percent called for in his healthcare policy's patient responsibility section.

Gerald's scrutiny of the $950 surgery bill led to a surprising discovery. Although insurance companies frequently complain about being duped by fraudulent policyholders and providers, Trigon and dozens of other health insurers and managed care companies stand accused of a scheme to siphon off millions of dollars from their policyholders.

How does the alleged scheme work? For surgery priced at $1,000, the typical plan might call for the insurer to pay 80 percent, or $800, which leaves the patient with a $200 copayment. But if the insurer has negotiated a 50 percent discount from the provider and does not pass any of the savings on to its policyholders, the patient's $200 copayment becomes 40 percent of the $500 actual bill, and the insurer's portion drops to only $300.

Trigon's responses to Gerald's queries stirred up more questions than answers. Norwood H. Davis, Trigon's CEO at the time, assured Gerald that he did indeed owe the $190 and added that the details of Trigon's provider contracts were "proprietary." In another letter, Norwood made a distinction between Trigon actually paying its $760 share of the bill and "discharging" it. Norwood added that although Trigon might try to persuade a provider to accept less than its $760 portion of the bill, a policyholder was free to do the same thing regarding the copayment. Gerald, who by that point was livid, replied, "Suggesting that an individual policyholder negotiate with a provider for price concessions borders on the insulting!" and threatened to take the matter up with state regulators.

At a time when consumers are expected to take more responsibility for their own healthcare, undisclosed discounts raise questions about the accuracy and honesty of information provided by insurers, providers, and employers. Indeed, providers often are contractually prohibited from disclosing discounts. The insurance industry argues that hiding discounts is not widespread, and Chicago-based Blue Cross and Blue Shield Association notes that no court has ruled for plaintiffs in a discounts-related case. It adds that none of its affiliates that settled such cases admitted to wrongdoing. Furthermore, Blue Cross and Blue Shield Association executives argue that the discounts benefit policyholders by reducing premiums and that some employers who share in the savings ask that discounts not be disclosed to their own employees. "We're not lining our pockets with anything because there is nothing to line our pockets with," said Joel Gimpel, a Blue Cross and Blue Shield Association attorney.

What do you think about the copayment problem? Does this case present an ethical issue? If so, to which party (or parties)? If you could act as the ultimate authority in this situation, what would you do?

DEAL OF A LIFETIME

CORPORATE-OWNED LIFE INSURANCE

2

Do you know what COLI stands for? The answer is *corporate-owned life insurance*. At one time, Wal-Mart was spending about $1 billion a year in premium payments to buy about $20 billion of life insurance coverage for 325,000 of its employees. Other big-name firms, such as Winn-Dixie, AT&T, Disney, GTE, Nestlé, and Procter & Gamble, have been doing the same thing. Some (or even many) for-profit health-care companies are probably doing the same thing, but no data are available to confirm this suspicion.

COLI, which is almost unknown outside of the insurance world, is sometimes called "janitors' insurance" to distinguish it from the life insurance that companies often take out on key executives to help offset their loss to the company from premature death and from corporate-provided life insurance that is part of a business's managerial fringe-benefit program. In fact, one corporate executive at Winn-Dixie was accused of calling COLI "dead peasants' insurance" in an interoffice memo. Needless to say, Winn-Dixie would not comment on the accusation. (The term *dead peasants' insurance* refers to the plot of Nikolai Gogol's novel *Dead Souls*.)

Here is an overview of how COLI works:

1. A company takes out, say, a $100,000 life insurance policy on one of its lower-level employees. The employee may or may not have to agree to the policy, depending on the state. If it is necessary to get employee approval, the company may offer to

231

pay a small amount—say, $5,000—to the family if the individual dies while an employee of the firm or $1,000 if the individual had left the firm prior to his or her death. This payment to the employee's family costs the employee nothing, so it is not hard to find willing participants when worker approval is required.

2. To pay for the policy, the company borrows the entire amount from the insurance company that issues the policy. Usually, the policies are single-premium policies, so only one up-front premium is paid. The company also borrows the money needed to make the interest payments on the policy loan, so no cash would flow from the employee's company to the insurance company while the policy is in force.

3. The company's bottom line is helped in two ways. First, increases in the paid-in cash value of the policy are reported as profits. Second, the company receives a tax-free death benefit when the employee dies, even if he or she has long ago left the company.

4. The company uses the tax-free death benefit to pay off the policy loan and to make the payment to the family, if one was promised, and then pockets the difference.

Most companies claim they use the money received from insurance benefits to pay for various employee and retiree benefit programs. However, this is very difficult to verify, and there is no requirement to do so. Furthermore, each dollar from COLI that is used for employee and retiree benefits frees another dollar to be used for executive compensation and perquisites.

What do you think about the concept of "dead peasants' insurance"? Does this case present an ethical issue? If so, to which party (or parties)? If you could act as the ultimate authority in this situation, what would you do?

BAYVIEW SURGERY CENTER

3

PRICING/BILLING OF SURGICAL SERVICES

JOYCE GRIFFIN IS an accountant who is also an avid tennis player. One fall afternoon, after an inspiring win at the tennis club, she noticed a sharp pain in her knee. The diagnosis was a torn tendon, which could be easily corrected by arthroscopic surgery. After consultation with an orthopedic surgeon whom she knew from the club, Joyce asked the physician to schedule the surgery for the following week at Bayview Surgery Center (the Center), a local ambulatory surgery center.

Being an accountant and detail minded, Joyce called the Center as soon as the surgery was scheduled to provide the required insurance information and to ascertain the amount of the charge. The patient accounts clerk at the Center quoted a charge of $1,500 for the surgery and told Joyce to bring a check for $300 the day of the surgery to cover the 20 percent copayment called for by her health insurance policy. Joyce paid the $300, and, fortunately, the surgery was a resounding success. In fact, Joyce was extremely pleased with the medical care provided by both the Center and the surgeon.

The problems began the following week when Joyce received a copy of the bill that was submitted to her insurance company. Her eyes almost popped out when she read the total—$2,657, which should have required a copayment of $531. Equally strange was that the insurance claim form showed no sign of her $300 copayment; the "Amount Paid" space had a zero. Confused by the inconsistencies between what she had been told earlier and the claims form, she confronted the Center's business manager for an explanation. The best answer she could get was, "This is just the way we do it. Everybody does it this way."

233

There are two ways of looking at this dual pricing of services. First, perhaps the Center is trying to give the patients—the "little guys"—a break; we might call this the "Robin Hood theory" of billing. Second, the Center might be trying to increase business by quoting a lower price to patients, and hence charging a lower copayment, but making up for the lower copayment by charging the insurance company more.

Neither of these possible explanations was very satisfying to Joyce, so she informed her insurance company and asked what it planned to do about the Center's pricing inconsistencies. But much to her shock and disappointment, her insurance company did not seem to care. Even worse, the letter she received contained these sentences: "We don't print money; we handle money. Do not worry about us overpaying for services because you, the consumer, through your employer, are ultimately paying for this."

What do you think about quoting one price for patients and another for insurers? Does this case present an ethical issue? If so, to which party (or parties)? If you could act as the ultimate authority in this situation, what would you do?

JEFFERSON GENERAL HOSPITAL

MERGERS, ACQUISITIONS, AND AGENCY

4

MARK MILLER, CEO of Jefferson General Hospital, has some tough decisions to make in the future. Jefferson General is a stand-alone, not-for-profit hospital that has a long and proud tradition of serving the community in which it operates. It was founded in the midst of the Great Depression as Jefferson County Hospital and remained under public control for more than 50 years. Then, in 1986, after years of losses, the county decided that it could no longer afford to operate the hospital, and it subsequently converted the hospital from a public to a private entity. At that time, Mark was brought in as the CEO. After a shaky start, he was able to turn the hospital into a moneymaker. Still, he was very aware of the hospital's roots, and he made sure that the hospital continued its original mission of providing healthcare services to the needy, regardless of their ability to pay.

Jefferson General is the smallest of the three hospitals that serve Jefferson and surrounding counties; the other two are St. Vincent's Hospital and Northwest Regional Medical Center. St. Vincent's has religious roots, but it is now operated as a not-for-profit, nonsectarian hospital. Northwest Regional is owned and operated by a large for-profit chain. The combined capacity of the three hospitals is more than 950 beds, but none of the three operates above 60 percent occupancy. Furthermore, managed care is starting to take hold locally, and hospital utilization trends indicate that the service area will need only 600 beds as utilization rates and the length of inpatient stays are squeezed down.

The most logical solution to the county's changing healthcare market conditions is a merger between two of the three hospitals, and

235

Jefferson General is the hospital most likely to be acquired. Mark has been approached by the CEOs of both St. Vincent's and Northwest Regional concerning his interest in a merger. Although it was too early to speculate on the exact terms that might result if a merger takes place, past mergers in the region provide some insights into what might happen to Mark should a merger occur.

If the hospital were acquired by St. Vincent's, Mark would probably continue as CEO of the hospital, at about the same compensation as he currently receives. However, he would lose much of his autonomy and authority because he would now have to report to the system CEO, who most likely would be the current CEO of St. Vincent's. Alternatively, if the hospital were acquired by Northwest Regional, Mark would probably relocate to a CEO position at some other not-for-profit hospital because the for-profit chain usually brings in its own management team when it makes an acquisition. But Mark would not go away empty-handed. He would probably receive a large "golden parachute" as a result of his job loss, which might include lucrative stock options, a lump sum payment, and a consulting contract. The aggregate amount of such payments could easily be worth many times his current annual salary.

Although the ultimate decision regarding the fate of Jefferson General rests in the hands of its board of trustees, the members of the board were chosen more on the basis of their community ties than on their business acumen. Thus, all those involved are aware that Mark's recommendations regarding the hospital's future will carry a great deal of weight in the final decision.

What do you think about the dilemma facing Mark Miller? Does this case present an ethical issue? If so, to which party (or parties)? If you could act as the ultimate authority in this situation, what would you do?

FRONT STREET HOSPITAL

5

UNINSURED CHARGES AND COLLECTIONS

WHO IS RICHARD "Dickie" Scruggs, and what does he have to do with hospital finance? You may not be familiar with the name, but you will undoubtedly read about his work and its influence on how uninsured patients are billed and the manner in which the bills are collected. You see, Dickie Scruggs ran a law firm in Pascagoula, Mississippi, that made huge amounts of money out of multibillion-dollar settlements from asbestos and tobacco companies. Then, his law firm turned its attention on the not-for-profit hospital industry. (To learn more about Dickie, both good and bad, and what he is doing now, search *Dickie Scruggs* on the web.)

In the early 2000's, his firm filed more than 70 lawsuits in federal courts against not-for-profit hospitals, alleging that the hospitals routinely overcharged self-pay patients, hounded them with aggressive collection tactics, and failed to provide adequate charity care in violation of their tax-exempt status. In a number of these lawsuits, the American Hospital Association (AHA) was named as a co-conspirator and defendant. Needless to say, the AHA called the lawsuits "baseless" and a diversion of resources that could otherwise be used for community healthcare.

At the heart of the lawsuits are two issues. First, the fact that patients who are least able to pay are generally charged the most. It is common practice to bill self-pay patients at full charges (chargemaster prices), whereas most every other payer is paying less than full charges, often substantially less. For example, consider the case of Jane Adams, age 22 and uninsured, who spent two days in not-for-profit Front Street Hospital for an appendectomy procedure. Her hospital bill was $14,000, and doctor's fees added another $5,000. It turns out that if a local HMO had insured Jane, the hospital bill would have been about $2,500. Medicaid would have paid about $5,000,

237

and Medicare would have paid about $7,800 for the same procedure. "Why do I get stuck with the whole bill?" asked Jane, "An uninsured person has a lot less money than insurance companies or government agencies."

Unfortunately, Jane stumbled onto a troubling fact of hospital finance: Most hospitals set official "charges" for their services but then agree to discount those charges for third-party payers. As a result, almost no one but the uninsured ever pays chargemaster prices. In some ways, hospital charges are like hotel "rack rates," which are posted prices that everybody knows nobody pays. But the hospital industry is different, because uninsured patients traditionally have been billed the equivalent of rack rates.

The second element of the lawsuits revolves around collection tactics. Although hospitals collect less than 5 percent of billings from indigent patients, many hospitals are very aggressive in their collection tactics. A press release announcing the lawsuits said that hospitals engage in business methods calculated to defeat the rights of uninsured patients. According to Scruggs, if and when the uninsured patient can't pay, not-for-profit hospitals often intimidate and harass uninsured patients through "goon-like and predatory collection tactics that frequently scar the patient for life, including the trauma of personal bankruptcy."

To illustrate, consider the case of Marlin Bushman, who was arrested, handcuffed, and taken to jail for missing a court hearing about a $579 Front Street bill. This collection tactic, known as "body attachment," has been abandoned by most other creditors. Said one observer, "The concept of debtor's prison as we understand it from Dickens' time is alive and well in the hospital industry." Another favorite strong-arm tactic is to place a lien on the patient's house. For example, Front Street placed a $3,600 lien on the house of Ben Pickett for a $3,000 unpaid hospital bill. Furthermore, a threat was made to foreclose on, and hence force Ben to sell, the house if the debt was not paid within 90 days. The interest on the debt was pegged at 12 percent, which means that Ben will never be able to pay it off because the interest is accruing faster than his ability to make payments.

The worst part of these billing and collection tactics, according to Scruggs, is that these policies are deliberately put in place to discourage the indigent from seeking healthcare services. By discouraging uninsured patients from seeking healthcare, not-for-profit hospitals are avoiding their obligation to provide charitable services as required by their not-for-profit status.

What do you think about the billing and collection policies of not-for-profit hospitals related to the uninsured? Does this case present an ethical issue? If so, to which party (or parties)? If you could act as the ultimate authority in this situation, what would you do?

WESTWOOD IMAGING CENTERS

6

PAYMENT FOR REFERRALS

MEDICAL IMAGING IS one of healthcare's fastest-growing sectors, so most everyone wants to get in on the action, including physicians. To illustrate, imaging costs are Medicare's fastest-growing service item. In recent years, they rose at three times the rate of other medical services, and the amount spent on imaging services has reached 15 percent of total healthcare costs. One reason for this rapid increase is the ability of imaging to detect conditions that previously required diagnostic surgery for detection. But another reason could be financial incentives that make some doctors order more scans than are medically necessary.

At a recent meeting of cardiologists, neurologists, and oncologists, Westwood Imaging Centers told doctors how they could get in on the boom. The deal works like this: Doctors would send patients to Westwood for imaging services, and Westwood would charge the referring physician a flat rate per scan. Then, the physician would bill the third-party payer for the scan at the going rate. For example, Westwood would charge physicians $375 for an MRI scan, while the average reimbursement for the scan is estimated at about $700. After deducting about $90 per scan for interpretation and administrative costs (mostly billing and collections), the profit per scan comes in at about $235 per referral. A group practice that refers ten patients a day would pocket about $600,000 annually under this plan. For more expensive PET (positron emission tomography) scans, the same volume would produce an annual profit for the referring group of more than $2 million. For the most part, the third-party payers would be unaware of the deal, assuming that the scans were conducted in the doctor's office.

But wait a minute, aren't such arrangements against the law? After all, federal antikickback (Stark) laws prohibit providers such as Westwood from paying doctors for referrals when Medicare or Medicaid patients are involved. These laws also extend to other types of patients under 36 state statutes. The Westwood plan also raises the issue of self-referral, which occurs when physicians refer patients to businesses in which they or relatives have a financial interest. When these prohibitions are considered, isn't the Westwood proposal illegal?

It turns out that there are exceptions to the antikickback and self-referral laws. One exception is that it is permissible to self-refer when the services are provided in the physician's office. For example, it is legal to order an electrocardiogram for a patient and then perform the procedure in the doctor's office. Clearly, the Westwood proposal does not meet the exception because the scans are done at Westwood's imaging center.

Westwood's solution to the legality issue is to characterize the scan not as a referral but rather as a "per use, nonrecurring lease agreement." In other words, when the scan is performed, the equipment and the space around it are "owned" by the referring physician, and hence the scan qualifies as a procedure performed in the doctor's office. Some imaging companies are using a slightly different approach. Instead of paying a charge for each scan, the physician (or group) books a set number of hours per week on a scanner, which they must pay for even if they don't send enough patients to use up all the time booked. This arrangement adds risk to the physician but supposedly is more resistant to antikickback laws.

Does anyone get hurt by such deals? Virtually all research done in this area indicates that utilization increases when doctors have a financial stake in providing imaging services. For example, one New York neurology practice with a lease deal ordered almost 50 percent more scans than did similar practices without such deals. It is hard to believe that the increased cost to insurers is medically justified, so the third-party payers (and ultimately the purchasers of health insurance) end up paying more than is necessary.

What do you think about Westwood's proposal to provide physicians with "leased" diagnostic equipment? Does this case present an ethical issue? If so, to which party (or parties)? If you could act as the ultimate authority in this situation, what would you do?

SPOTLIGHT ON PODS

PHYSICIAN-OWNED DISTRIBUTORSHIPS

7

ACCORDING TO THE American Academy of Orthopaedic Surgeons (AAOS), there were almost 28,000 orthopedic surgeons practicing in the United States in 2013. Many of the procedures performed by these surgeons involve spinal, hip, or knee replacements, which require medical device implants that cost close to $15 billion per year.

In recent years, there has been a trend in the industry toward physician-owned distributorships (PODs), which now account for about 25 percent of all sales of orthopedic devices. The concept of a POD is simple: Physicians (mostly orthopedic surgeons) team up with nonmedical personnel (usually sales agents or other distributors who are already selling the devices) to form a new business. This new entity (the POD) purchases products directly from manufacturers at what is commonly called a "transfer price," which is far lower than the list price or even the prices offered to hospitals and other end users. The POD then sells those same devices to hospitals at a markup, which may be substantial, over its costs. This approach is a traditional stocking distributor model with one twist: The physician-owners of the POD are also the ones ordering and implanting the devices.

During a panel discussion at the 2011 AAOS Annual Meeting, representatives from government and device manufacturers joined orthopedic surgeons in reviewing the pros and cons of this distribution model. Here are some of the views presented.

According to one California orthopedic surgeon who has ownership interest in a POD and in device companies, surgeon-owned distribution systems are "a model whose time has come." In his view, physician

241

ownership encourages volume pricing, controls costs, and fosters competition. Where PODs have been introduced, he noted, substantial cost savings have resulted. PODs provide the orthopedic surgeon the control necessary to compete in an accountable care organization (ACO) and bundled payment environment. It's a great ancillary business that provides value to hospitals and society, he said.

The surgeon then explained that PODs negotiate with manufacturers and agree to purchase in bulk and to assume the financial burden of inventory. The POD replaces distributors, who, he argued, add very little to the value of the implant. Salaries for product representatives are more in line with those paid to other healthcare providers, such as nurses and physician assistants, and the difference is distributed to the providers (surgeons and hospitals) of the service. He also discussed the American Association of Surgeon Distributors (AASD), a trade association that was recently established. The goal of AASD is to establish a set of standards governing the legal and ethical use of the surgeon-owned distribution model and to gain endorsement of these standards by the government.

Conversely, another panelist, a staff member of a prominent US senator, noted that several congressional inquiries into PODs have been launched, although Congress has not taken any official position on the subject. She expressed concern about the impact of PODs on medical decision making; in her opinion, the proposed models for these systems need close scrutiny to ensure that the potential for financial inducements does not affect medical decisions.

PODs, she noted, are prevalent in the fields of spinal surgery and total joint replacement and are increasing in the field of cardiology—all areas in which Medicare spends substantial dollars. Initial investigations found that some PODs distributed a great deal of money to physicians who had made just a small investment, limited their business only to investors, guaranteed high returns on investment, and ensured that more surgeries were being performed by surgeon-owners. These issues all raised concerns with members of Congress and resulted in additional investigations. "Not everyone is a bad actor," she admitted, "but we believe these models deserve close scrutiny."

What do you think about PODs? Is it alright for surgeons to profit from prescribing certain implants or for hospitals to protect referrals by sourcing through PODs? Does this case present an ethical issue? If so, to which party (or parties)? If you could act as the ultimate authority in this situation, what would you do?

About the Authors

Louis C. Gapenski, PhD, is a professor of health services administration at the University of Florida. He is the author or coauthor of more than 20 textbooks on corporate and healthcare finance. Dr. Gapenski's books are used worldwide, with Canadian and international editions as well as translations into Bulgarian, Chinese, French, Indonesian, Italian, Polish, Portuguese, Russian, and Spanish. In addition, he has published more than 40 journal articles related to corporate and healthcare finance.

Dr. Gapenski is an active member of the Association of University Programs in Health Administration and the Healthcare Financial Management Association and is a Faculty Associate of the American College of Healthcare Executives. He has acted as academic adviser, chaired sessions, and presented papers at numerous national meetings. Additionally, Dr. Gapenski has served as an editorial board member and reviewer for 12 academic and professional journals.

George H. Pink, PhD, is the Humana Distinguished Professor in the Department of Health Policy and Management, Gillings School of Global Public Health, at the University of North Carolina at Chapel Hill and is a senior research fellow at the Cecil G. Sheps Center for Health Services Research at the university. Prior to receiving a doctorate in corporate finance, he spent ten years in health services management, planning, and consulting.

Dr. Pink teaches courses in healthcare finance and is involved in several large research projects, including studies of hospital financial performance. In the past 20 years, he has served on the boards and committees of more than 100 hospitals and other healthcare organizations. He has written more than 70 peer-reviewed articles and has made more than 200 presentations in ten countries.